I0058057

# The Low Back Pain Guide

Answers To The Most Common Questions About
Diagnosis, Treatment Options, and Spine Surgery

**DR. GEORGE M. GHOBRIAL, M.D.**

The Low Back Pain Guide

Copyright © 2019 by George M. Ghobrial, M.D.

All rights reserved. No part of this book may be reproduced in any form or by any electronic or mechanical means, including information storage and retrieval systems, without permission in writing from the publisher, except by reviewers, who may quote brief passages in a review. This book may not be reproduced, copied, transmitted, or stored in part or in whole, without the written consent of the author. The information in this book is not meant to represent or serve as a substitute for medical care. The data contained herein is meant for educational purposes. This book does not serve as a warranty or guarantee of the completeness or accuracy of this information. The content presented in this book is not a substitute for medical care by a physician, and should not be used for self-diagnosis, primary medical advice, or medical treatment.

ISBN 978-1-949148-01-5 (Paperback Edition)
Library of Congress Control Number 2019908174

llustrations by Aaron Hoover of Mountain of Strength, LLC.

Editing by George M. Ghobrial, M.D.

Printed and Bound in USA
First Edition First Printing July 2019

Published by Weatherly Press
Spine Team Six, LLC
P.O. Box 536
Pfafftown, NC, USA 27040

*For Michelle,*

*Alexander, Nicholas, and Timothy*

# Preface

Largely due to the internet, a wealth of information is readily available to most people- millions of books, videos, and other media are available at any time. This has certainly been the case for healthcare where the internet serves as an abundant source of immediate information for any medical question that a patient may have. The internet can teach anybody about any general or obscure topic of interest, which includes medicine. Someone can be educated by watching lectures, reading articles written by 'experts', connect with other people with similar goals, and even obtain rare and out of print sources of literature on a subject, previously only available at universities and large libraries.

With healthcare information, two challenges stand out.

The first challenge is sorting the information into material that is relevent from information that is irrelevant or unhelpful. The second challenge is even harder, which is to gain a sense of the quality of the information. No two sources of information are equal. While you would take advice from a community message board in order to troubleshoot software problems on your computer, it is a risky venture to do the same for back pain.

Your personal health is not like your other hobbies, and so there is a limit as to what you should do on your own when it comes to self-directing your medical care. These boundaries will be discussed throughout this guide to low back pain. The singular message carried throughout this book is to seek help from and discuss your healthcare decisions with a healthcare provider in whom that you have developed trust.

Patient education is important- being fully informed alleviates anxiety and can help everyone make smarter healthcare decisions. In order for this book to be most helpful for the reader, it is organized as a reference material. It is a collection of common questions frequently asked by patients with low back pain. It is organized into five sections, in a chronological order. The first section is an introduction on the topic of low back pain, followed by a guide to early back pain pain management, followed by a primer on understanding spinal imaging and tests, and finally a concise assessment of the available treatment options which can includes surgical or early medical treatments(nonsurgical).

The most common questions can be found in each section. For example, a patient recently had an MRI of the lumbar spine. They read their report, but did not understand the description by the radiologist. In this book, these terms and common imaging questions relating to the significance of these findings are located in section III. This reference is complete with straightforward illustrations when necessary.

This book was designed for anyone to be able to pick up and use. It will not assume that you have any prior medical training. It is not possible to go over every topic in this book in great detail, as it would be thousands of pages and encompass numerous medical specialties. Instead, this book will help you understand modern back pain management and get pain relief in a clear and direct manner!

# Introduction

Low back pain is one of the most common medical problems face everyone in their lives, regardless of your health,
fitness level, occupation, or status in society. At any given
time, more than 15% of people report that they have low
back pain (LBP). In fact, this is so common that it is referred to as part of *the human experience.*

Why is it so common? There are numerous causes of low
back pain. Modern technology has allowed us to expand
the list of problems that cause LBP using innovative ways to
diagnose and treat LBP. Often, there is more than one cause

of low back pain. Further uncertainty is raised since we do not fully understand the numerous causes of LBP. Often, You may not be able to determine the exact cause of your low back pain.

In this book, from the perspective of an expert in the field of low back pain, we will discuss the most common causes of LBP that are both related to the spine and even frequent causes that are not coming from the spine. As a neurosurgeon who helps patients deal with low back pain, the author has organized this book into a list of some of the most common questions that are encountered in a clinic.

Since then, the healthcare experience today is rapidly becoming more patient driven, and the healthcare market is starting to resemble a consumer marketplace. Consider the following example. Your car breaks down on your way to work. You miss work that day and go to a mechanic. Eventually, a mechanic explains the problem. He also identifies a few problems along the way, then describes several systems including breaking, transmission, and suspension. He then talks about parts, labor, and the time they need to complete the job.

First, your health is so much more important than a car. The stakes are so much higher and there are no nonmedical analogies that appropriately capture the emotions that you would be going through if you had to miss work and seek professional help for low back pain. However, there are several clear similarities. Returning to the car example, there is pressure to make a decision without understanding what exactly is going on, there usually is a high financial cost, and there is significant pressure to make a decision. The pressure comes can come from the low back pain, your desire for pain relief, and your need to be independent- in order to return to work.

Outside of healthcare, having to make major decisions

with financial implications is becoming more common, and on more highly technical subjects. We will see more and more scenarios like these as we further integrate these technologies into our lives.

While the same holds true with medicine, the stakes are so much higher when the decision applies to your health or the health of those you love. Healthcare is rapidly getting more complex and more confusing.

This book is an attempt to demystify low back pain for you, but it is not a do-it-yourself manual. Just like you would not replace the brakes on the family minivan used daily by your wife and kids, just the same for your low back. This book is recommend that you use this book as a helpful reference, but only in tandem with advice and consultation from an expert in the medical field.

The process of obtaining healthcare is rapidly specializing more and more, and it involves more and more appointments. At times, some patients have not had time to fully digest all of the information at each appointment as well as the purpose of some visits; The road to LBP relief is not very straightforward. When would it be an appropriate time to accelerate your workup for a diagnosis of LBP? When is it appropriate to obtain imaging? Once the imaging is obtained, what do patients do next? Patients are torn between numerous treatment options, medication, alternative medicine, treatment such as spinal injections, and ultimately all of the surgical treatment options. This book will address these questions.

Imaging reports are more commonly available to patients for review, and certainly create confusion due to the long and cryptic description used to describe the spine. Most patients arrive in the neurosurgical clinic with just a basic understanding that low back pain is due to pain coming from the spine. Often, they bring with them their MRI, or magnetic resonance imaging (MRI) study that give a highly detailed picture of the spine (or anywhere of relevance for other medical specialties). A radiologist is a doctor who carefully analyzes the MRI and provide a description/report. Some of the questions that you may ask yourself that are ansered in the imaging section are among the most frequent: Are all findings a cause of LBP? Are they all a sign of disease, or a sign of the aging process? If these findings correlate with pain, do the findings correlate to your pain? How does my treatment relate to this finding? Does it mask these symptoms of the underlying problem? Or, does it correct the underlying problem? Getting an imaging study may very well unlock the path to some of the most expensive and invasive surgical and nonsurgical treatments. These options are discussed in this book.

For most flare-ups of low back pain, the pain will improve without any form of treatment. Depending on the severity and your daily demands, perhaps you can hold off a little while longer for imaging, and see if there is improvement.

Regardless, your adventure will be unique, and not all circumstances can be controlled, regardless of how much research you do. Educate yourself about the treatment options for low back pain, including those presented in this book, and carefully consider all of your options and see how this fits You. Any treatment recommendation should be tailored to fit your unique lifestyle, values, and understand what your goals and expectations are before undertaking any therapy. Most of your education will be web-based and I will lay out some general principles to help you be cautious in how you get your online information about spine health.

-George M. Ghobrial, M.D.

# Contents

# III: SPINE IMAGING EXPLAINED

# IV: NON-SURGICAL TREATMENT

# V: SURGICAL TREATMENT

# Section I

# Getting Answers

# 1  What is low back pain?

Low back pain (LBP) is a discomfort centered below the ribcage, centered over an area called the lumbar spine, commonly involving the muscles, nerves, ligaments, and bones of your back.

The primary focus of low back pain in this book is the spine, althought we will discuss later in the book the numerous causes of low back pain other than the spine. The spine is the primary support structure of your body that keeps you upright (your 'backbone') and is comprised of blocks of bone called *vertebral bodies*, which are the building blocks of the spine. The spine also protects the spinal cord, which is a bundle of nerves that allows the brain to receive sensory information and sends signals to control  your limbs, perceives pain and other sensations, helps control your bowel and bladder functioning, and also helps control and organize other vital systems (ie. Organs, blood vessels, skin, etc...).

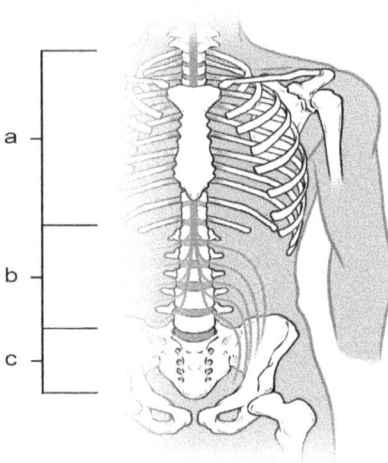

*The spine consists of seven cervical segments (vertebrae, not shown), and typically carries nerves to and from the upper extremities. The thoracic spine (a) is twelve segments, and are connected to the twelve pairs of ribs. This is the least common region to be affected by degenerative disc disease due to the limited flexibility and limited motion that occurs here. (b) The lumbar spine is five levels and carries nerves down to the lower extremities. This region is the most common area to be affected by painful problems of disc degeneration due to the increased motion and bearing the weight of the majority of the body. (c) – The sacral spine does not contain mobile discs and is where five pairs of sacral nerves travel through to the pelvis and lower extremities in the case of S1.*

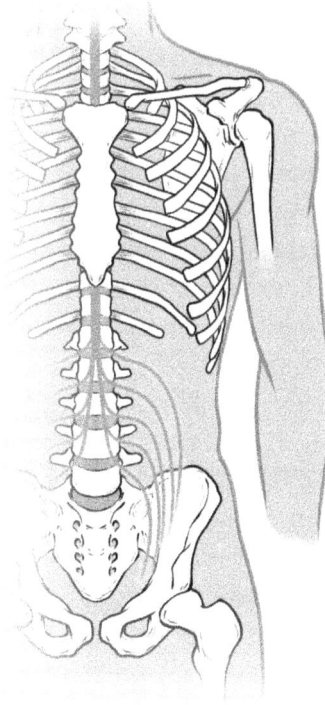

*The spine consists of the vertebra, which are blocks of bone and are separated by intervertebral discs. They allow for an upright posture and locomotion. The spinal cord (center line) runs to and from the brain, down the spinal canal. Segments of nerves exit at each level in the neural foramen, which are spaces between joints at each level that serves as entrances and exits for nerve roots.*

In between the vertical stack of vertebral bodies are shock absorbing cushions called *intervertebral discs*, or *discs*. The structure of the spine gives us our upright posture and the discs are the flexible shock absorbers of the body, that provides flexibility. The discs are made up mostly of water, collagen, and interface with the bone of the vertebrae above and below with a surface.

Low back pain is the second most common reason to miss work and accounts for a fifth of all claims for work-related injury. This problem affects most adults in our society. It is in fact the most common reason to go into the doctor's office to seek medical attention.

It would be impossible to go through life without experiencing back pain at some point. Some experience this pain worse than others. Since LBP is so common, it makes sense to take the necessary steps to inform yourself about your options and preventative measures to reduce LBP without professional help. This book is a great start for that. Many patients that seen in the clinic seek immediate pain relief from urgent care, emergency rooms, and family practice offices at the immediate onset of LBP. I will be discussing later in the book some of the many things that can be done on your own that can help with LBP. Often, once someone is already caught up in the routine of weekly professional care and treatment of LBP, which includes visits to healthcare professionals and daily medication, they often forget that there are many simple things that they can do that have profound effects on low back pain. There is a growing list of acceptable noninvasive therapies not discussed in this book, and in order to keep this reference concise, a limited number of options are described.

## 2  How Common is Low Back Pain?

Low Back Pain is the most common health problem that an adult will experience, and often results in pain and disability. LBP is becoming more common. In a study performed in North Carolina, the incidence of chronic LBP increased from 3.9% in 1992 to 10.2% in 2006. Also, the likelihood that patients with chronic LBP would seek medical attention from a healthcare provider also increased. In fact, up to 84% of adults have LBP at some point in their lives. One out of every four adults in surveys report in the last three months that they've had an episode of LBP. This high disease prevalence carries overwhelming costs. In fact, the cost of caring for LBP in a single year for US patients was estimated to be $100 billion in 2006 both due to direct and indirect costs. Indirect costs add to a large expense, which is due to lost productivity, and lost wages.

# 3    What Causes Low Back Pain?

Low back pain is caused by a number of structures that interact with the spine to provide motion: muscle, ligaments, joints, pelvis, sacrum, nerves, and other soft tissues. The most common cause has been identified as the lumbar disc (diagram below). This is referred to as discogenic low back pain.

The spine will age over time, or degenerate, contributing to back pain. This is a slow process of degeneration and it affects multiple components. This is not much unlike a car, which eventually will require replacement of the shocks, struts, breaks, tires, etc... (hopefully not much else). Unfortunately, at the present time, none of the components of your spine can be swapped out like a car. Pain coming from the discs is termed *discogenic pain*, which is thought to be the most common cause of LBP in younger patients. The older you are, the more likely that the facet joints are contributing to your overall LBP. Probably the most significant factor in developing LBP is just time, as the process of aging of the spine or degeneration, is a time-dependent process affecting all mobile joints.

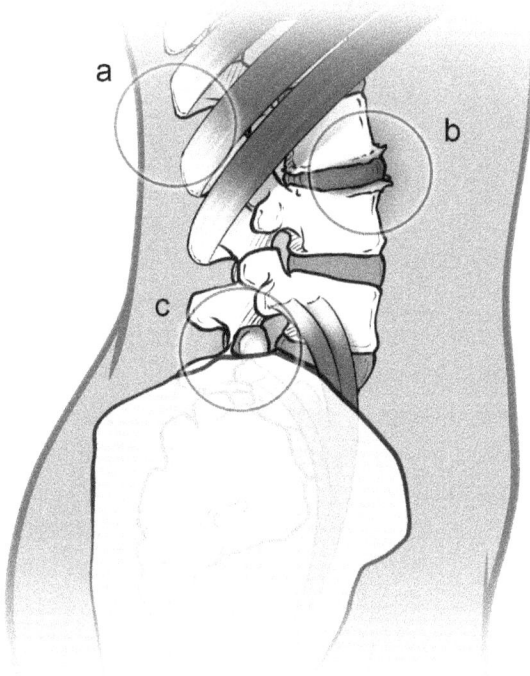

*Common causes of Low back pain. A- muscles and ligaments: Normal life predisposes us to the eventual onset of painful muscle sprains and strained ligaments. This heals slowly, and is a common cause of chronic back pain B- Discogenic pain can bring about painful inflammation. While the term degenerative disc disease is a common MRI diagnosis, it is often in people without pain. It can affect multiple levels and is difficult to confirm as a cause of pain. C-Facet- Each level of the spine contains a left and right facet joint, which is involved in stabilizing the spine and providing flexibility- its degeneration can cause LBP.*

# Discogenic Pain

## A KEY CONCEPT OF SPINAL AGING

The discs age over time. As the discs age, they dehydrate, and lose the volume that provides shock absorption and flexibility. Dehydration may cause cracks to form in the posterior lining of the disc(a radiologist may call it an annular fissure in an MRI report). This lining is called the *annulus fibrosus*, and separates the disc from the spinal canal, where the nerves course. As the discs degenerate, increased pressure on the adjacent bone causes painful inflammation resulting in low back pain (discogenic pain).

Other changes are occuring with less disc material to absorb forces of gravity on our spine. Increased stress applies to the bone surrounding the disc, and the joints behind it. This principle was first described in 1892 by Julius Wolff, a German surgeon. He identified that the more weight you put on a bone surface/joint, the more dense that bone becomes. The bone will then spread out to increase the surface area to lower the overall pressure on the surface(which is force divided by the area). In the spine, each block of bone has cartilage above and below, with a special joint filled with water and a jelly-like protein called collagen, and all of this makes up the disc. No matter what, over time, the disc dries out. This may not occur at the same speed for everyone.

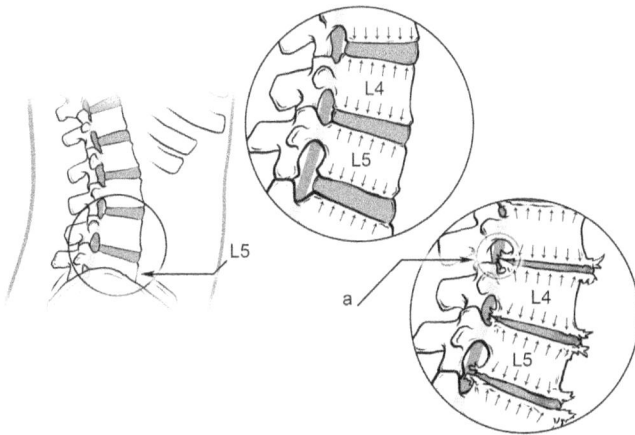

Degenerative Disc Disease(DDD): Although present in the majority of adults over 40, the loss of water in the disc results (center image) in shortening of the disc and decreased room for the exiting nerve. Increased motion will occur at the level where a disc shortens. Bone spurs form which are areas of new bone growth in attempts to increase spinal stability, along with thickening of the ligaments, and arthritis of the facet joints which can either decrease the room for the nerves ( arrow *a*, right image) and cause nerve compression, or cause painful spinal joint pain.

*DEGENERATIVE DISC DISEASE*

*Degenerative disc disease*(DDD) is a term originally used to describe the painful inflammation that degeneration of the discs brings about. This is thought to be the cause of 39% of LBP! However, DDD has come to be a very common imaging diagnosis in people without symptoms. Just because they call it a disease does not make it a problem that necessarily requires aggressive treatment. This is one of the most common concerns with patients entering the office.

### DISCOGRAPHY- CAN IT IDENTIFY THE PAINFUL DISC?

If most LBP is caused by discogenic LBP, can discography, a study to identify a painful disc be useful? Discography is a procedure where a needle is guided into the center of a particular disc space with the intent to reproduce or increase the pain intensity. Since this procedure itself has been shown to create painful discogenic pain in people without prior discogenic-type pain, it has fallen out of favor with many clinicians due to mixed reviews. How does the disc generate pain? The outer layer of the disc, called the annulus, has pain fibers, which can increase in number with chronic inflammation. Keep in mind that not all abnormal discs are painful!

## Myofascial Pain

Muscles and tendons in your back can easily become overloaded and cause LBP. This type of pain will go away with rest. Serious strains and sprains are slow to heal. More serious injury to the muscle can result in shortening or scarring of the muscle, which can feel like firm, tender, nodules. Many doctors offer trigger point injections of long-acting anti-inflammatory medications into these painful areas providing excellent relief.

## Facet Joint Pain

The joints in the lumbar spine can generate pain as well. These are called facet joints. LBP that is worse while standing, laying flat, or other positions with the back extended, such as carrying of heavy loads can contribute to facet joint pain. This pain can be worse when walking down stairs or twisting.

## Spinal Stenosis and Neurogenic Claudication

Conditions causing crowding and pressure on the nerve roots in the spinal canal can cause LBP as well as leg pain and cramping. This leg pain and cramping is often termed neurogenic claudication, and accompanied with an intense pressure in the low back. When you lean forward, the ligaments in your spinal canal may stretch providing just enough additional room to decompress the nerve roots and provide some relief in symptoms. This symptom is a hallmark of spinal stenosis. In medicine, stenosis is a common term which generally means narrowing of a passageway. This narrowing is usually caused by degeneration of the spine and growth in the bones and ligaments, resulting in crowding of the nerves. This process takes most of your life and commonly is an issue requiring treatment in your sixties and later. Part of the population is born with less room for the nerves, due to a smaller spinal canal. With less room to accomodate this crowding, symptomatic stenosis happens earlier, and this is often referred to as congenital spinal stenosis. This could occur as early as in the thirties and fourties, and is accelerated by additional lifestyle factors such as obesity and smoking.

## Piriformis Syndrome

The sciatic nerve is a bundle of nerves that travels down the legs, compression of which causes painful sciatica. This begins with tenderness and a focal area in the buttock and can mimic low lumbar spinal pain. This is often seen in sedentary people and prolonged sitting can cause low back pain and pain that travels down the back of the leg. Piriformis syndrome is a separate issue, thought to be a major cause of LBP and leg pain.  As the sciatic nerve exits the pelvis and travels down the back of the leg, a small muscle in close proximity, the piriformis muscle, can potentially compress and irritate the sciatic nerve as it travels around the muscle en route to the leg.

## Sacro-iliac Joint Disease

Sacroiliac(SI) joint disease is another cause of low back pain that receives less attention. The SI joint is a large joint space articulating between the sacrum(part of your spine) with the pelvis. The diagnosis of an SI joint disease in a primary care office by examination alone of the SI joint is not straightforward. SI joint pain can be described as a sharp, dull, achy, or cramping pain overlying the buttocks. Occasionally, sharp pain can radiate down the posterior thigh, and terminating before the knee. One possible indicator of SI Joint disease is where a provider has you lay down on your back, and hang your leg over the edge of the bed- If this is painful, causing discomfort in the small of your back and off to one side, this could be an indicator of an SI joint problem.

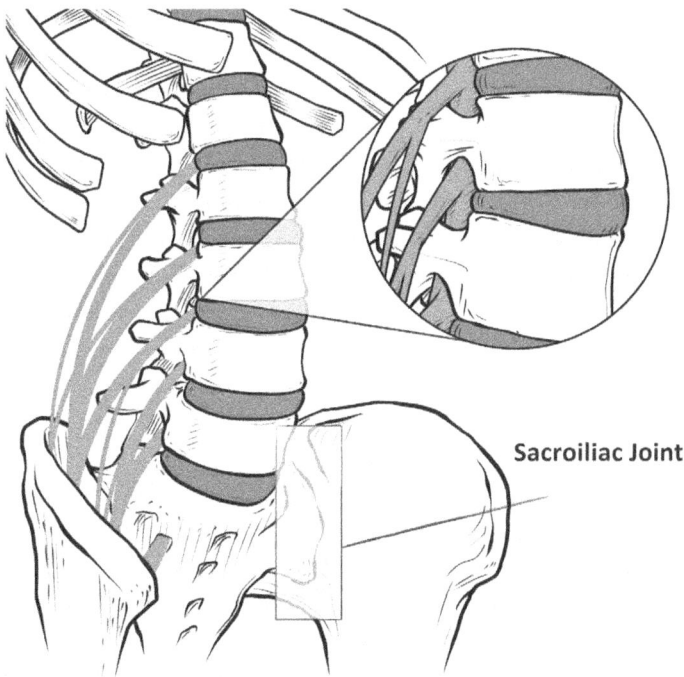

*Sacroiliac Joint – Located to the right and the the left of the sacrum. This is a vertical joint where the spine meets the pelvis. It is thought to be a common joint driving low back pain.*

| Common Causes of Low Back Pain Due to Degenerative Disorders of the Spine ||
|---|---|
| Discogenic Pain | Inflammation of the Disc |
| Mysofascial Pain | Muscle sprains and strained ligaments resulting in abnormal pain. |
| Facet Joint Pain | Athritis of the paired joints of your spine. |
| Spinal Stenosis With Neurogenic Claudication | Symptomatic nerve root crowding in the central spinal canal which causes low back pain, leg pain, and a relief with bending forward. |
| Sacro-iliac Joint Pain | A large joint at the interface of the pelvis with the sacrum, which causes back pain and leg pain. |

# 4 Why Do I Have Pain Shooting Down My

# Leg(Sciatica)?

At each level of the lumbar spine, a pair of nerve roots exits the spine through openings called the *neural foramen*. The nerves then travel down to your legs to provide motor control and nerves also carry sensory information such as touch, temperature, position, and pain the opposite direction to the brain for processing.

The sciatic nerve is the largest nerve in your body, and is made up of the fourth and fifth lumbar, and first sacral nerve roots. These nerves join up outside of the spine, and are called the sciatic nerve which courses down the leg branching into smaller nerves that innervate muscles in the legs and feet. The most common term for pain shooting down the leg has been called *sciatica*, which is generally a term used for any pain radiating down the leg.

## THE NERVE ROOT EXITS THE SPINE IN CLOSE PROXIMITY TO THE NORMAL DISC

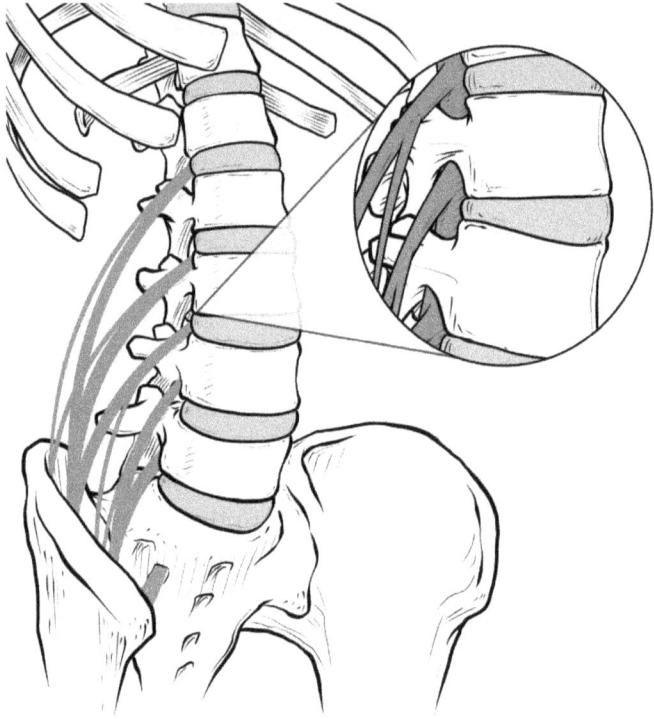

*At each level of the spine, a pair of nerves exit. The exiting nerve is in close proximity to the disc space, where disc herniations can compress the exiting nerve, called the neural foramen. The nerves exit and some join into larger nerves. The sciatic nerve is a combination of nerve roots from L4, L5, and S1 nerves.*

Usually, nerve pain travelling down the leg that is true sciatica continues past the knee. The nerve root irritation occurs at the level of the spine, before they join to become the sciatic nerve. The term lumbar radiculopathy is used to describe compression or irritation of the nerve root before it exits or while exiting the lumbar spine. Another term for radiculopathy is dysfunction of a nerve root which is associated with pain, sensory impairment, weakness, or decreased reflexes associated with the distribution of that nerve.

There are other causes of radiating leg pain that can mimic irritation of the lumbar and sacral nerves that travel down the legs. These could include problems with the hips, pelvis, and sacroiliac joint(SI joint). The SI joint connects the pelvis to the sacrum, a nonmobile region of the spine(it has no discs). Discogenic LBP can also cause painful symptoms in the legs that do not follow a typical pattern similar to nerve root irritation.

## DERMATOMES- NERVE ROOT FUNCTIONS ARE SPECIFIC

In the lumbar spine, a pair of right and left nerve roots exit each level and eventually reach a consistent region of the skin, or a specific group of muscles. A dermatome is a specific region where a known nerve root provides sensation. This region is fairly consistent from person to person. For example, sensation to the skin on your heel is typically supplied by the S1 nerve root. As a result, maps have been made and are provided freely on the web showing this pattern of nerve root coverage for sensation. If you had numbness over the front of the thigh, it may indicate an L2 nerve root region.

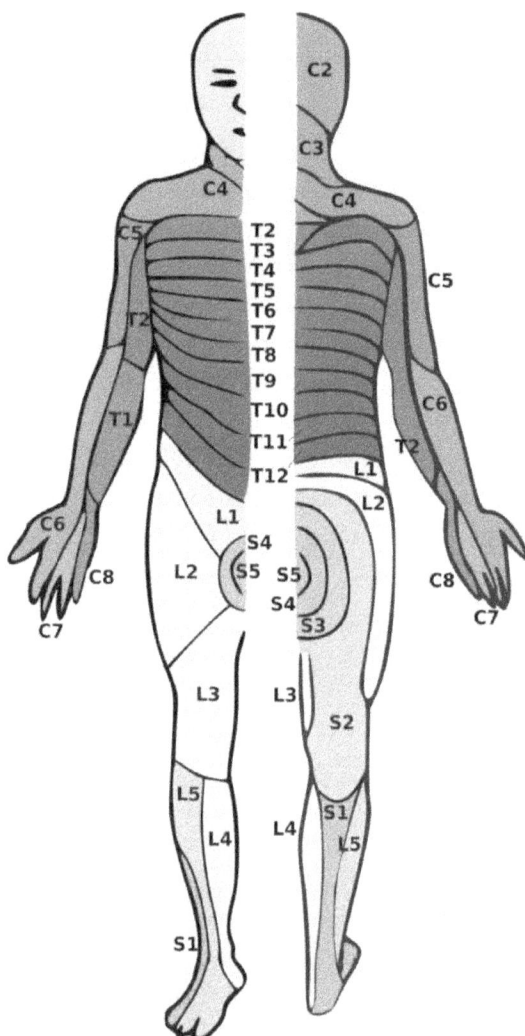

*Map of the dermatome (image from public domain). This diagram represents the areas of the body where sensation is supplied by correlating nerve roots which convey sensory information from the skin to the brain.*

## WHY ARE THESE MAPS SLIGHTLY DIFFERENT ?

Interestingly, there is a variation to some degree on where the nerves run down the legs and what precise locations each nerve goes to. This is thought to be due to discrepancies with how we number the levels of the spine and very slight variations in anatomy between people. Usually the differences are slight, but it adds to the challenges with identifying the cause of painful nerve root compression.

A color-coded illustration of the front and back of the body correlating to where the nerves are expected to supply is called a dermatomal map with labels for different nerve root levels that carry sensation. When you look at one web source versus the next, the location of various nerve distributions differ. These is likely due to the occasional variation seen between one patient to the next.

# 5  What Are Some of the Spinal and

# Non-Spinal Causes of Low Back Pain?

There are numerous causes of low back pain. It is not important that you learn how to diagnose and impossible for you to self-diagnose your cause of LBP. You will need the help of a medical professional. However, along with the previous chapters about types of low back pain generators, a few key points can help you expedite your care and raise your level of understanding :

# Key Points

- Most often acute back pain flare-ups are musculoskel-etal, which means it could be pain coming from one of the many small muscles that attach to the bones of your spine. There are numerous small muscles along with the tendons that attach the muscle to the bones of the spine, and small ligaments that the bones of one vertebrae to the neck. These structures are subjected to constant daily stress. Overuse of the muscles causes acute muscle strain, which ranges from overstretching of a muscle to tears of the muscle. Sprains involve stretch or tear injuries to the ligaments. Ligaments in the lumbar spine are very tough, designed to withstand a high degree of tension, and will not completely tear, except in the case of major trauma. Strains and sprains are usually a source of chronic back pain and are the focus of many non-invasive back pain treatments, including stretching, physical therapy, and chiropracter treatment.

- One common cause is a disc herniation – A recent disc herniation can cause severe LBP, and this is very common. This causes leg pain too! The location of the disc herniation plays a role in that.

- Most importantly, a recurring theme in this book is that an imaging study is more likely than not to diagnose a condition of the spine. This doesn't mean it is causing a problem, or your current painful symptom, or any symptom. This is where a spinal expert can help you go through the diagnostic process and guide you through the process at getting better.

# Spinal Causes of Low Back Pain

By far the most common cause of low back pain begins with the degeneration of the disk, a natural process of aging. Other less common causes of LBP related to the spine could include benign and malignant tumors of the spine, spinal infection, osteoporotic compression fractures, scoliosis, muscular strains and ligamentous sprains that results in inflammation and back pain.

# Non-Spinal Causes of Low Back Pain

Perhaps least well-known by patients coming into the office is that visceral diseases, that is, certain abdominal problems can cause chronic low back pain. These could be the harbinger of a serious health condition. These include kidney stones/nephrolithiasis, prostate problems, gallbladder stones/cholecystolithiasis, aortic aneurysms, urinary tract infection, and pelvic inflammatory disease. Essentially, any disease that impacts nerve fibers that carry pain signals to the brain can give a pattern of symptoms that includes low back pain. Metabolic diseases can impact the bones and cause back pain or even spinal fracture. Although the most common cause of low back pain is of musculoskeletal origin, there are so many diseases that share low back pain as a symptom, the work up and medical care absolutely needs to be done under the care of a healthcare provider such as your physician.

## NONSPINAL CAUSES OF LOW BACK PAIN AND PAIN PROCESSING/PSYCHOLOGICAL DISTRESS

Stress and depression may manifest as low back pain. Psychological stress in our lives, anxiety-provoking events, personal loss, major depression, and posttraumatic stress disorder, are examples of a few psychological problems that influence pain processing. Studies have shown that people with more severe depression are twice as likely to have LBP at the 4-year follow-up interval. Persistent low back pain has been linked with the diagnosis of depression and anxiety. Untreated depression decreases the likelihood of a successful surgery.

## 6 How long does Low Back Pain Last?

Low back pain is described as the human experience. This means that it is impossible to go through life, without episodes of transient back pain. For back pain caused by a flare-up due to a disc herniation, or inflammation from musculoskeletal causes, most episodes resolve in 3 months. To some degree, improvement occurs with or without professional help. Moreover, in 19 out of 20 patients, leg and back pain decreases substantially or resolves within the first 3 months. In fact, of the 95% of people that experienced the first onset of leg pain, most observed a dramatic relief and symptom intensity over three months. This is why many healthcare providers state that most people do not require surgery. However, whether it does go away or not without seeing a care provider depends on many factors, and without knowing the actual cause, it is hard to predict exactly what will happen for each person. The bottom line is, getting medical care often takes time, and this time can be all that you need to experience resolution in pain.

# SECTION II

# EARLY BACK PAIN MANAGEMENT

27

## 7    When Should I Be Concerned About

## Low Back Pain?

It is not uncommon today for patients with the first time onset of low back pain to seek immediate treatment either from their primary care doctor, urgent care office, chiropractor, or emergency department. While the majority of medical problems are related to common degenerative conditions of the spine, some associated symptoms or known medical issues may warrant a more urgent medical workup under the direction of a healthcare provider. While there is no definite rule encompassing all scenarios, there are a number of general findings either from past medical, surgical, social history, and symptoms of yours that may constitute a "Red Flag Conditions".

Red flags are physical exam findings and signs(detected

by the physican), or symptoms, or a history suggestive of an increased probability of having an underlying urgent medical problem,  or any neurologic symptoms / injury which could influence initial treatment.

While there is considerable debate over the value of some of these conditions in terms of predicting underlying medical problems that require an urgent evaluation from a healthcare provider, the American College of Physicians and the American Pain Society published a few red flag conditions. For example, one example would be someone with a history of cancer and now they have new low back pain symptoms- see your physician immediately for further advice as one possibility is that there is a spread of the cancer to the spine(or neighboring anatomy).  In this scenario, since there are too many variables to discuss, such as recent remission, known tumor in your spine, or recent radiation and chemotherapy and radiation treatment, or recent surgery for cancer.  Regardless, new LBP should be communicated promptly to your oncologist and they can determine the best treatment at that point.

| |
|---|
| **MEDICAL HISTORY RAISING URGENCY TO SEEK MEDICAL ADVICE FOR LOW BACK PAIN** |
| - History of cancer |
| - Intravenous drug use/recreational drug abuse |
| - Weight loss |
| - Recurrent urinary tract infection |
| - Fevers |
| - Bowel or bladder incontinence/dysfunction |
| - Trouble walking /balance problems |
| - Muscle weakness |
| **CONCERNING PHYSICAL EXAM FINDINGS IN THE SETTING OF LOW BACK PAIN** |
| - Decreased sensation in the groin/saddle area |
| - Motor weakness |

# When To Get Help Early:
# Summary Recommendations

The American College of Physicians proposed recommendations on when to get an MRI for nonspecific low back pain without leg pain. If at any time there is some concern, seeking immediate medical help is the best course of action:

- History of cancer- makes cancer a possible presenting symptom of low back pain. Discuss this with your physician

- Previous history of cancer and/or, elevated markers of inflammation (ESR. CBC), or weight loss

- Risk factors for spinal infection such as fever, history of recent infection, history of drug use

- Concern for cauda equina syndrome: new urinary retention, incontinence, back pain, and/or changes of sensation in the groin/perianal area(numbness)

- Prior spinal surgery

- Known spinal condition AND new or worsening symptoms

## 8  What Can I Do Immediately For the

## Pain?

The good news is, there are many options to get you out of pain. Many societies recommend avoiding any invasive therapies or advanced imaging such as an MRI for the first 3 months, if at all possible. Often, spinal pain is relentless and debilitating, and the process of obtaining a diagnosis and treatment increases the liklihood the patient will be presented with more invasive treatments within the first three months.

WHY WOULD MEDICAL SOCIETIES GUIDE PHYSICIANS
TO AVOID INVASIVE TREATMENTS AND ADVANCED
IMAGING IN THE FIRST 3 MONTHS?

The answer is that first time flare-ups of low back and leg pain improve regardless of treatment intervention over the first 3 months. If possible, providers are encouraged to limit prescribing of controlled substances and especially to avoid potentially harmful medications(such as addictive opiate medications) and other invasive treatments.

Summary of American College of Physicians General Recommendations for Acute Low Back Pain(2017)

- In the 2017 guidelines by the American College of Physicians: physicians are urged to avoid prescribing medications for acute low back pain(<4 weeks), which can include opioids, steroids, tricyclic antidepressants, and selective serotonin reuptake inhibitors(SSRIs).

- Often the pain is very severe limited most daily activity. If patients see their doctor, it would be preferred to start with a nonsteroidal anti-inflammatory drugs(NSAIDS) or skeletal muscle relaxants.

- Also, within the first four weeks, massage, acupuncture, or spinal manipulation therapy(chiropracters) are reasonable options for pain relief.

- After 12 weeks, pharmacotherapy with nonsteroidal anti-inflammatory drugs, tramadol, or duloxetine is reasonable. Tramadol is a controlled substance and is addicting.

- Opioids are only an option if these other medications have failed. These are a last resort medication.

## WHAT CAN I DO IF I HAVE PAIN THAT TRAVELS DOWN MY LEGS?

The recommendations are the same, favoring the least invasive of treatments, regardless of the addition of leg pain. Leg pain can often be far worse than low back pain, and is described as sharper, brief, episodic, and electric shock-like. Howevere, due to the lack of high-quality medical studies that show any additional benefit from invasive testing and treatments, most societies urge that these are avoided.

Moreover, the North American Spine Society, a group of medical professionals with the goal for evidenced-based, high-quality spinal care, recommends the least aggressive management of lumbar disc herniations with radiculopathy within three months of onset. They concluded that the majority of patients improve, regardless of treatment. This is more than likely because most disc herniations shrink and regress to the point that they are no longer compressing nerve roots over time.

## 9 Where Can I Get Help, and Where is the First Place To Go?

There is no absolute answer to this question. Since most flare-ups of back pain resolve spontaneously, and in line with the 2017 guidelines by the American College of Physicians(ACP), you want to go somewhere that can provide pain relief in a conservative manner (the least invasive way possible). This is usually a primary care office, but there are often more convenient locations(discussed in question 10) where the same treatment can be obtained.

## 10   What are the Differences Between Urgent Care, the Emergency Department, and My Primary Care Office?

Episodes of Low Back Pain that are initially evaluated in an urgent setting end up being triaged and referred to an outpatient clinic setting, which in some regions leads to an appointment several weeks later. There are three very common locations for back pain to be evaluated, and that includes an urgent care clinic(acute care clinic), the hospital emergency department, and a primary care office(outpatient clinic).

# Emergency Department

The emergency department(ED) should be avoided for acute low back pain without 'red flag conditions', if at all possible. The ED was not designed to handle back pain, the most common reason for an adult to go to the primary care office. The time it takes to be seen by a healthcare provider after entering the ED is the longest of the three options, and this is because patients with life-threatening conditions are steadily entering the ED and being prioritized for care(a process called triage). There are numerous dynamics at play in the ED and many historical, social, and economic factors that make the ED the worst option for most episodes of acute LBP.

Another consideration with entering the ED is that the cost of care is much higher than if you were to get the treatment in the urgent care or primary care clinic. There are many reasons for this, but the two main reasons are that there is a greater likelihood that you will obtain more expensive imaging studies and medications, and that the costs are higher in the ED due to the higher cost of resources in a hospital setting.

Trauma and acute low back pain is one instance where an emergency department is the most reasonable setting for an evaluation, however. For the most part, unless you are unable to carry out basic daily activities such as walking and self-care(eg. eating and getting dressed), an urgent care clinic, primary care clinic, or other specialist clinic would be a more appropriate setting for seeking initial care.

# Urgent Care Clinic

Urgent(almost emergent) care clinics arose out of a need for cost-effective and efficient care options for common painful conditions. Urgent care clinics are excellent for painful low back pain requiring same-day attention. Examples of conditions commonly requiring urgent attention (as advertised on websites from various urgent care clinics) include: a cut that may require stitches, but does not have significant bleeding, sprains, strains, and back pain.

# Primary Care Clinic

As mentioned in several other areas of this handbook, primary care clinics handle the most common patient complaint next to the common cold- which is low back pain. The physicians and providers in the primary care clinic are experts at appopriate evidenced-based treatment. This means that you are less likely to end up with second and third line treatments and advanced imaging upfront. This includes lumbar MRIs, injections, and controlled substance prescriptions. Recalling the 2017 American College of Physicians Guidelines, the goal is to avoid as much treatment as possible in the first three months, since back pain typically subsides within three months.

Another advantage of the primary care clinic is that

preauthorization is more likely to be obtained for imaging studies, referrals, and advanced tests and treatments. Some insurance companies are denying coverage of these expensive and invasive diagnostic tests in the first three months. Keep this in mind, that if you go to the ED and an MRI is recommended, your insurance may not cover it.

One last point to keep in mind with primary care clinics is that you have the chance to obtain care for a problem that will more than likely require follow-up for, and unlike in an urgent or emergent setting, in the clinic you have the opportunity to go over your treatment options with a physcian or provider who you have developed a relationship with.

# 11  What Can a Pain Management Doctor

# Do For Me?

A pain management team resides in a clinic, like a primary care office, except they focus exclusively on acute and chronic pain and can provide the widest range of available treatment options in the office. This office has  the greatest expertise to tailor pain treatments to each individual.

There are several considerations regarding if a pain management team is needed.  Historically, chronic pain treatment included long term use of prescription medications, with a high likelihood that opiates were integral to that treatment.  Due to the increase in opiate-related deaths, chronic opiate treatment is being avoided.  Increased regulation regarding opiate prescriptions as well have led to the effect of increased referrals of patients with chronic back pain to be sent to pain specialists for primarily the chronic management of opiates.

## Pain Management Considerations

A pain management office is most like a clinic setting and requires an appointment. Typically, this is not an urgent care clinic where you can be seen without an appointment (called a walk-in). While acute pain can be treated, the approach will be similar to the American College of Physicians 2017 guidelines. Multiple visits may often be required as well. Develop a relationship with the provider that you are most comfortable with. Call and discuss what therapies are offered before scheduling and waiting for an appointment. Some offices do not offer certain interventional procedures and some offices have restrictions regarding pain management.

### COMMON PAIN MANAGEMENT SERVICES

- Assess patients to help diagnose causes of spinal pain: low back pain and leg pain can be difficult to distinguish due to similarities in pain caused by the hip, pelvis, SI joint, lumbosacral nerves, and spine.
- Prescribe medications that relieve acute and chronic pain in line with evidenced-based guidelines.
- Provide targetted injections with pain relieving medication into the spine.

- Some pain management physicians provide evaluations for spinal cord stimulation (see section, spinal cord stimulation).

The pain management physician and his/her team specializes in the short and long term treatment of pain, offering a comprehensive diagnostic and treatment program for a particular problem. The modern standard is a fellowship-trained pain specialist. Fellowship training is additional training completed after residency, which is completed after graduating residency.

The American College of Graduate Medical Education recognizes three board certifications in pain treatment- those are the american board of anesthiology, american board of psychiatry and neurology, and the american board of physical medicine and rehabilitation.   Understanding a provider's overall philosophy of pain management, especially in spinal pain management, is very important, because for chronic low back pain a long term doctor-patient relationship may be established, and you want someone that you are comfortable with and with similar treatment goals.

Often, an initial evaluation may not be with a pain management doctor, but rather with an nurse practitioner or physician assistant on the team. These team members are closely supervised and carefully trained by the pain manangement physician and allow the physician to have you seen as early as possible. Since there are so many people with back pain seeking care by a pain management doctor, this arrangement allows for you to be seen in a reasonable amount of time.

Occasionally, patients are wary of pain management clinics, and that stems from the misconception that these clinics primarily treat pain with opiate prescriptions.  To the contrary, opiates (eg. Hydrocodone, oxycodone) represent a very small component of treating spinal pain because they are ineffective, and have a high addiction potential and other side effects.

Pain management doctors are the most appropriate referral for initial nonsurgical care of a patient with a degenerative spinal disorder, due to the wider range of appropriate therapies that they can provide from their office. Whereas, in a surgeon's clinic, the main tool of treatment is surgery, which is only needed by a fraction of patients. Often, some clinics are organized so that pain management doctors will establish your treatment plan, and for patients that end up needing surgery, they see the surgeon who is part of the same multispecialty clinic.

Commonly, for severe and disabling pain not alleviated by medications, a pain management physician can provide injections of medication into the spine, which are guided by x-rays and delivered precisely aroujnd the inflamed nerve. This provides higher concentrations of steroids, anti-inflammatory medication, or analgesic medication to the area that is needed- which explains why an injection can be so much more helpful for patients than oral medications.

Oral medications are less potent because they can be distributed throughout the body, potentially causing more negative side-effects. These injections a versatile, and in addition to injections around the nerve, they can be injected into numerous joint capsules at a site of suspected pain, and superficially into the muscles. The degree of pain relief may be helpful in patients with suspected pain coming from multiple sources, as it helps physicians understand all of the causes of pain in a particular person. Many pain management physicians provide a number of other targeted treatments, called interventional pain treatments, which will be discussed in the upcoming section on non-surgical treatments.

## 12    What Can a Physical Therapist Do For

## Me?

The majority of acute low back pain is due to musculoskele-tal causes.  As a result, the best initial treatment is daily and consistent stretching, core strengthening, and other con-ditioning exercises.  This is the least invasive treatment for acute low back pain and arguably should be utilized more than it currently is.  Physical therapists and their staff help with core strengthening, which is a great way to improve posture, and improve overall quality life.  In some studies, patients with acute low back pain who were referred to physical therapy for 8-12 weeks were less likely to require advanced spinal imaging or further testing.  One rationale for this protocol and a partial explanation why this protocol works is that it required patients to wait 3 months.  As we have discussed, most acute episodes of low back pain will go away without intervention during 3 months.  Overall, physical pherapy is a good initial therapy for acute low back pain.This is because of how safe it is. It carries a fraction of the risks that have been reported with some other therapies.

## Are There Any Particular Physical Therapists That Specialize in Spinal Conditions?

For the most part, there are self-designated spine subspecialists among the physical therapy centers.  However, it is rare to fnd a physical therapists exclusively seeing spinal patients.  Physical Therapists trained in 'mechanical diagnosis and therapy' or the McKenzie Method (M.D.T.)  are exceptionally helpful, which is a speciality certification.  This is a speciality treatment process that works for localizing pain caused by most musculoskeletal problems.

However, most physical therapists can provide safe and helpful care for You. (see question 39 for more details). Your inital appointment is much like a doctor's initial care visit, where over the course of approximately 45 minutes you will meet with a physical therapist.  The physical therapist helps you by listening to your medical problems, assessing your overall medical wellness, makes an assessment to determine what the underlying cause is, and creates a plan for you.  This plan outlines all the treatments that you need, how often you will need them, and how long your course of therapy will be.  There may or may not be a follow-up appointment to reassess your progress. In some practices, your time spent with a physical therapist will be limited, due to the high demand. You will be more than likely spending your time with a physical therapy assistant(PTA), who will guide you through each step of your session. The PTA will help you go through the prescribed treatments appropriately, and safely. This is important for the spine to prevent injury.

## 13  What Can a Chiropractor Do For Me?

A chiropractor provides spinal manipulation and other manual treatments such as traction (chiropractic medicine) to relieve pressure on the nerve roots.  Spinal manipulation therapy(SMT) is another term for treatment provided by a chiropracter that is specific to the spine.  It may be defined as manual therapy, mobilization, and/or maneuvers that have the goal of relieving spinal nerve compression and ultimately relieving sciatica and/or low back pain.

HOW WELL DOES THIS WORK?

The mechanism of how physical therapy and SMT alleviates pain from a disc herniation is least understood by patients.  However, several studies have attempted to summarize the effects of SMT and to determine how well it reduces pain. One such study, a meta-analysis, is a study that attempted to summarize all of the available studies (a scientific way of finding a consensus for a specific question about a treatment, with the data coming from numerous, smaller studies), with the goal to analyze the effectiveness of SMT at reducing low back pain. It was concluded that SMT is beneficial for 'greater than 50%' of patients, in other words, you are 'more likely than not' to find a benefit earlier on.

Medical research regarding the helpfulness of SMT is difficult to adapt to real life, regardless of the conclusion that the majority of patients benfit from SMT. Other considerations are that this study does not take into account the issues of how often you have to go, how long the benefitof SMT will last(the pain reduction), and how helpful is it in the long term. However, the cost is far less than invasive medical treatments and many prescription medications, which is why several insurance companies will pay for this treatment as well as physical therapy.

In summary, like most initial treatments for acute low back pain, this is a good option for low back pain treatment early on because the risk profile is low, and for some people it can be useful in decreasing the likelihood that you will proceed down the line and obtain spinal treatments that are more invasive.

## 14 What Are the Differences In Spinal Care Between an Orthopedic Surgeon and Neurosurgeon?

Overall, for the majority of degenerative spinal conditions that require spinal surgery, there is no difference between an orthopedic surgeon and a neurosurgeon that could impact the outcome of your care. Nearly all surgical problems that stem from the degenerative disorders of the spine (disc herniations included) can equally be treated by either specialty. Today, the management of spinal disorders has become so complex that many surgeons undertake an additional year after residency where they complete a 'fellowship training' in spine surgery. This is an additional year of training after residency.

Today, most orthopedic surgeons that do not have fellowship training will not practice spinal surgery or be credentialled by a hospital due to a limited exposure to spinal surgery during residency. Spinal surgery comprises a greater portion of neurosurgery resident education, and for the most part, most neurosurgeons consider themselves capable in the surgical care of routine spinal problems. Overall, it makes no difference whether the surgeon is a neurosurgeon or orthopedic surgeon when it comes to the most common spinal problems.

## DIFFERENCES IN TRAINING FOR LESS COMMON SPINAL PROBLEMS

Some spinal problems requiring microsurgery are treated more often by a neurosurgeon, as the tools and techniques for some surgeries are common to the handing of microin-struments and nerve tissue. The spinal cord has a leathery covering that holds in all of the cerebrospinal fluid, called the dura. For spinal diseases that require crossing this barrier, ie. opening the dura to operate on the spinal cord, a neurosurgeon typically handles this. Again, this is a fraction of spinal problems and out of the scope of the low back pain guide. The overwhelming majority of spinal diseases are treated by either specialty, and each surgeon's unique training gives each and every surgeon a unique perspective.

Moreover, AOSpine Europe, a European Academy of spinal surgery research and clinical care, issued a 60 question quiz to each of its 289 responding members(spinal surgeons), and they found no significant difference in the test knowledge between neurosurgeons and orthopedic surgeons with regard to the management of spinal surgery problems. One-third of all respondents completed an additional one year subspecialty training in spinal surgery.

HOW A POST-RESIDENCY FELLOWSHIP IN SPINAL
SURGERY CAN BE HELPFUL

There is one area identified within spinal surgery that
it may benefit the patient to seek care from a fellowship
trained surgeon.  Scoliosis and spinal deformity(abnormal
and symptomatic malalignment of the spine) affects all ages.
Due to the extent of surgery often required and the relatively higher risks of complications, surgeons that completed a
one-year fellowship demonstrated on testing a significantly
greater knowledge base in the area of deformity surgery
compared to spinal surgeons not trained in spinal deformity.

While knowledge base does not translate into surgical
skills, surgical planning is critical in spinal deformity surgery.  Spinal deformity includes scoliosis and abnormalities
in the curvature of the spine which requires fusion across
large regions of the spine. Surgical treatment is among the
most technical challenges and the likelihood of a complication is the highest. Understanding the appopriate periop-
erative care for these patients can mean all the difference
in achieving a positive outcome.  Similarly, in the United
States, orthopedic spinal surgeons were tested on their
knowledge of spinal deformity surgery where it was shown
that of the 413 surgeons that responded, fellowship training
correlated to a higher score.

In summary, no major training differences could be de-
termined with surveys between neurosurgeons and orthopedic surgeons in a North American Study and if you have a
degenerative spinal condition, you are in more than capable
hands irrespective of which office that you choose to go to.

## 15    What Are the Roles of the Spine

## Surgeon When It Comes to Low Back Pain?

The traditional role of the spine surgeon is to evaluate a patient for spinal surgery. However, many spinal surgeons, like other spine specialists, will evaluate patients with acute pain, to help them obtain rapid pain relief.

The majority of disc herniations and episodes of low back pain and leg pain will spontaneously improve without intervention. Often, some spinal problems may cause severe and disabling pain despite most nonsurgical therapies. For a number of other reasons as well, at the discretion of your primary care physician, a patient may be referred to a spinal surgeon for an evaluation in their clinic for surgery. While this can be anxiety provoking, often patients are referred to spinal surgeons by their primary care physician because they are more comfortable with a spinal surgeon that they have developed a positive relation with to facilitate the discussion around recently obtained imaging.

This is very common and a referral to a surgeon in this instance and may not always mean that there is a concern that surgery is needed.

| **List of Common Services Offered by Your Spine Surgeon in the community:** |
| --- |
| Urgent evaluation for acute low back or leg pain, assistance with diagnosis and treatment |
| Surgical treatments: discectomy, nerve decompression, spinal fusion. |
| Referral for physical therapy |
| Minimally-invasive surgical options |
| Epidural steroid injections |
| Other targeted pain injections |
| Spinal cord stimulation |
| Vertebroplasty |
| Surgical treatment - nerve decompression |

# SPINE IMAGING EXPLAINED

# 16   Should I Get Imaging (X-ray, CT, or MRI)?

For most people with acute low back pain, diagnostic imaging is not required. In fact, all major medical societies relevant to the care of the spine have published position statements discouraging the practice of obtaining an MRI for routine acute LBP.

As mentioned in the 'red flags' section, imaging may be necessary in the event of weakness, difficulty walking, abnormal bowel or bladder function, trauma, osteoporosis, a history of cancer, LBP that is worse at night, fever, and ongoing treatment for an active infection or a history of recreational drug abuse. The most appropriate imaging study is often a lumbar x-ray, which can be helpful as a screening tool, but it is most often quickly followed by an MRI, as the x-ray does not show soft tissue well and is not as useful as an MRI for degenerative disorders of the spine.

Any decision making to obtain imaging requires a prescription by a primary care provider. The same goes for an MRI which obtains the highest level of detailed imaging of the spine. MRIs are essential for diagnosing nerve compression, but not necessary for most patients.

If at all possible, and you have not met any 'red flag conditions' it is important to avoid obtaining an MRI in the first three months. MRIs in adults almost always have some finding. In the face of acute LBP, it makes this finding hard to ignore, and it is hard to convince yourself that just because there is a "finding" on an MRI, doesn't mean it is causing your pain! In some instances, some studies are required to confirm that these findings are relevent.

One research study performed by an orthopedic spinal surgeon, identified a very high frequency of a spinal degenerative condition being diagnosed by an MRI obtained on a volunteer. These volunteers did not have symptoms, and were only 20-39 years old- more than 30% of participants had degenerated discs and more than 20% had disc hernations(not causing symptoms).

# When to Consider Urgent Imaging

Urgent imaging may be considered in the presence of weakness, balance issues, decline in bowel or bladder function, and numbness in your groin, fevers, recent trauma, chest pain, abdominal pain, or severe pain causing an inability to move.

Just like we discussed, You should seek medical help and obtain a more detailed medical workup if you have any of these Additional Symptoms(Red Flag Symptoms):

- fevers
- weight loss
- numbness
- weakness
- balance problems
- walking trouble

If You do not have any of these above conditions:

You do not need advanced imaging right away. Low back pain is common. Most back pain is short-lived and goes away without treatment during the first 3 months.

## 17    When Should I Get X-Rays?

X-rays use radiation, which is emitted through your body, and ultimately captured on film, creating the imaging study. The combination of unique anatomy, varying tissue density and composition, and decades of research and study of common appearances of normal anatomy and abnormal problems, the x-ray study can provide enormously useful information.  However, since most of the painful conditions of the spine are due to conditions related to soft tissues, x-rays are of little benefit.  X-rays are also limited in their evaluation of fractures as well, especially in osteoporotic patients where the clarity of small fractures may not appear all to well on an x-ray.  Since an x-ray only  provides a 2-dimensional picture on a flat x-ray film, atleast two x-rays shot 90 degrees apart are required to get a sense of the three-dimensional nature of the problem.

X-rays still have their place in spinal care, but as an intial test, they have limitations. They are still very useful as a screening tool to evaluate someone's spinal alignment and test for scoliosis as well as evaluate a patient with a past spinal surgery, and many other specific conditions. Additionally, they are inexpensive and easy enough to be obtained periodically through time to evaluate for any chronic changes that may be occurring.

Of the studies, they are the least expensive to obtain and frequently do not require prior approval to obtain and are found in imaging centers in many practices.

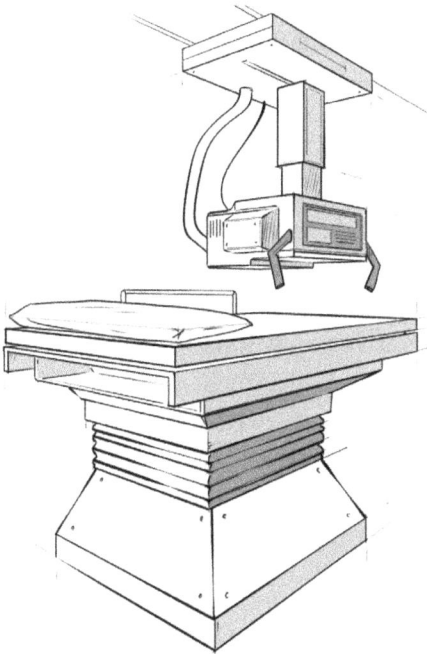

*X-ray machine, artist illustration. Obtaining X-rays may involve a special table, where x-ray film is placed underneath the body region for the examination. Radiation passes through lower density tissue in greater amounts, producing a picture.*

## 18 **When Should I Get a CT ?**

A CT scan(computed tomography) is less commonly required in the treatment of degenerative conditions of the spine for early-onset Low Back Pain. There are some less common degenerative conditions where a spinal surgeon may wish to obtain a CT, but most often, an MRI is the preferred imaging study to be obtained. CT scans are most helpful for evaluating fractures, calcified disc herniations, and other problems pertaining to the bone, which best shows up on a CT (compared to an MRI).

## What is a CT scan going to show?

CT scans also relies on radiation and can be used to obtain 3-dimensional imaging, whereas x-rays produce a 2-dimensional evaluation.

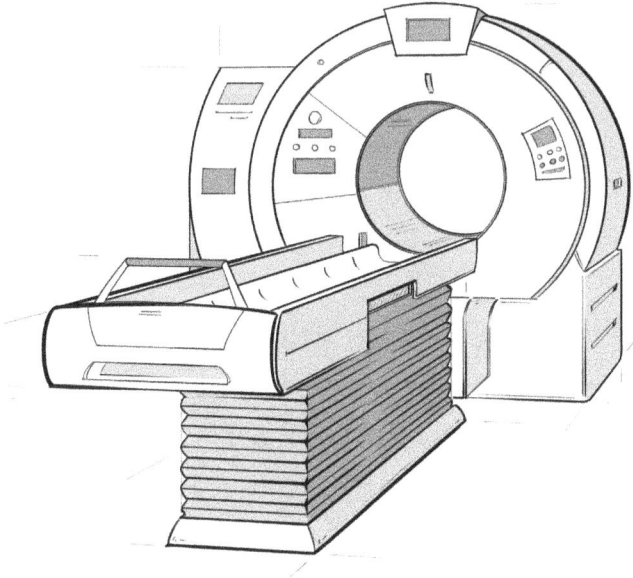

*CT-scanner, artist illustration. The scans involve briefly passing through the center of the scanner, taking less than a few minutes (in contrast to an MRI, which takes minutes to hours).*

## 19 **What is an MRI(Magnetic resonance imaging)?**

An MRI (Magnetic resonance imaging) is an imaging technique that uses a large electromagnet to provide the most detailed study of the body. MRIs do not rely on radiation. A powerful MRI can temporarily align positive charges (protons) in the body. Since water concentrations vary throughout the body, when the MRI aligns the charges, radiowaves are pulsed through the body to put the protons out of alignment. The time for the protons to realign with the magnetic field and any energy released varies by the tissue type. Refinements to the technique over time have allowed for very detailed anatomical pictures of the spine to be obtained.

Relative disc degeneration can be evaluated best by MRI. For example, as a disc degenerates, it loses water, which has a uniquely different signal than a healthy, hydrated disc. Another example is the condition of the spinal cord, where spinal cord inflammation is a seriously condition.  Previously this could not be detected with any other imaging study. Inflammation is a process of abnormal blood vessel permeability, where water will increased in the region of inflammation, which accounts for why a bruise becomes enlarged. MRI is particularly sensative to inflammation.

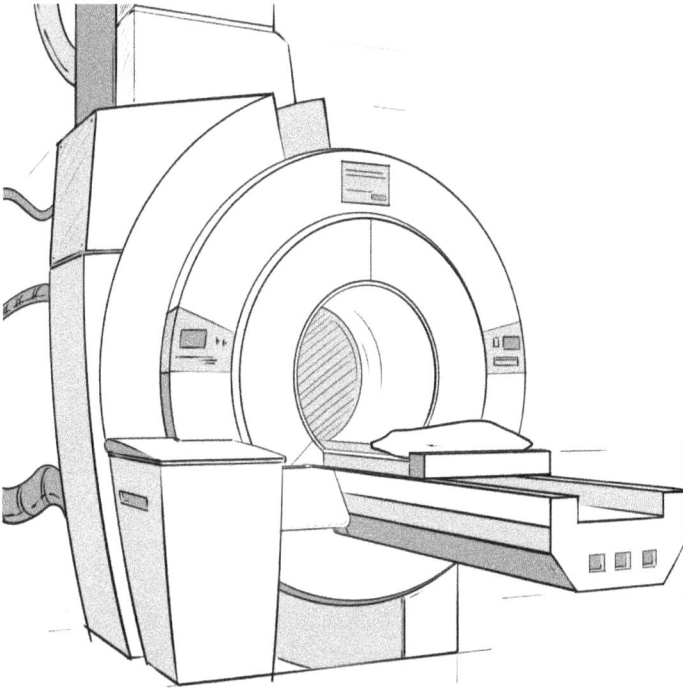

*MRI scanner. The Mri scanning bed retracts into a more confined space for a period of minutes to hours. The MRI scanner is loud, and patients typically wear headphones. For patients with difficulty in confined spaces, this may often require some type of mild sedation.*

## 20 How Can I Better Understand My MRI Report?

It may be a very difficult task to truly understand an MRI, however, with the trend of providing patients with digital access to their healthcare records, one common issue is being presented with data that appears concerning and diffi-cult to piece together.

It is important to realize that most people will not be able to understand their MRI report. Below is a list of common MRI terminology to help you better understand your MRI report.

## 21 **When Should I Get an MRI?**

An MRI is not commonly required for acute low back pain. Since most back pain episodes improve spontaneously, many insurance companies require additional treatments to be attempted prior to obtianing an MRI. Most often, a primary care provider will evaluate you first, to evaluate you for concerning conditions that warrant an early MRI.

## MRI Reports and Disc Bulges

That all depends on where the disc herniation is located and where your pain is located. Just remember, there are no absolutes! This is because everyone is wired differently, there are many causes of sudden onset pain, and a provider with experience can help you put this all together.

| My disc her-niation is often located: | My pain is commonly found to radi-ate(refer to the dermatome diagram): |
|---|---|
| L1-L2 | into my groin, across the front of my body. |
| L2-L3 | into the front of my thigh, terminat-ing above my knee. |
| L3-L4 | Across my outer thigh, and over to my knee. |
| L4-L5 | Down the outside of my leg to my ankle. |
| L5-S1 | Down to the top of my foot, crossing over to my big toe |
| L5-S1, but af-fecting the S1 nerve root below | Down the buttock back of the thigh, back of the knee, back of the calf, to the sole of the foot, affecting the outside of the foot. |

## What Are The Strengths of an MRI?

This is what you obtain when you are looking for the majority of problems in the spine. MRIs are helpful for disc disease and are the single most important study for the diagnosis and evaluation of a herniated disc.

## What if I Can't Obtain an MRI ?

In the case where you can't obtain an MRI, say for example, you have a medical device implanted, such as a pace-maker, then you can obtain a CT myelogram. A CT my-elogram (figure) provides a detailed picture of spinal canal compression. First Contrast dye is injected during a lumbar spinal puncture, which is a sterile procedure performed by a physician on a CT scanner table. The contrast mixes with spinal fluid, and then flows up the sac which contains the neves and spinal cord and will travel up the spine in the di-rection of the brain if the table is tilted with the head below the body. Compression on the sac from external sources, such as from discs, stenosis, etc., will easily show up on these studies.

**Comparison of Three Imaging Techniques: X-ray, CT, and MRI**

| Test | Im-plants | Radia-tion | Duration of Test | General diagnostic use | Expense |
|---|---|---|---|---|---|
| X-ray | Yes | Yes | Minutes | Fracture, scoliosis, spondylolisthesis, spinal infection, and other conditions with involvement of the bone. | $ |
| CT | Yes | Yes[1] | Minutes | Fracture, severe trauma, pars fracture, spondylolisthesis Evaluation of prior spinal hardware and the bone after previous surgery. | $$ |
| MRI | ★ [2] | None | Variable, often greater than 1 hour | Disc herniations, extent of stenosis, tumors, infection, epidural hematoma, spinal cord compression, spinal cord diseases, nerve root diseases, any nerve or spinal cord compression, ligament injury | $$$ |

1     *A CT uses multiple x-rays to create a more complex picture.*

2     *Radiologist approval required.*

## 22    What is Degenerative Disc Disease?

Despite how commonplace this term is, it is debated by many people as disc degeneration is thought to be a natural process of aging. And if the majority of people have it, then it is less of a disease and more of a natural process.  Others assume that degenerative disc disease (DDD) in the context of healthcare is DDD causing symptoms.

As you get older, the content of water decreases in the disc. The disc loses volume and eventually loses height. Inflammation can set in at the junctions of the disc and bone above and below, causing inflammatory changes in the endplate.

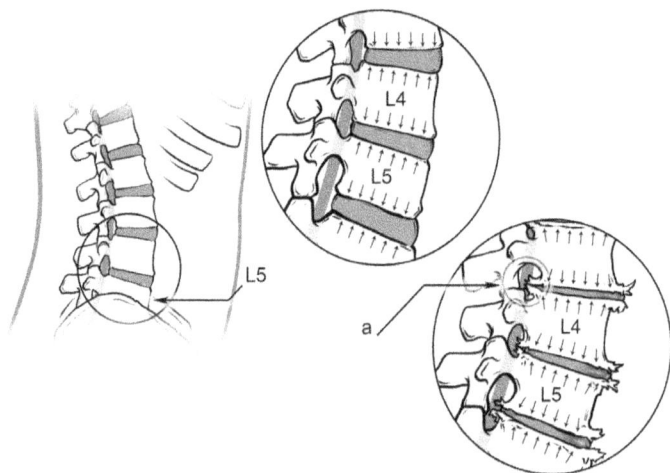

*Degenerative Disc Disease – A natural process where the disc material shrinks over time, resulting in increased motion. The body responds to increased motion resulting in potentially symptomatic inflammation and arthritis.*

## 23   What is a Disc Herniation?

The intervertebral disc is a shock absorber located between each segment of bone in the thoracic and lumbar spine. Segments, called vertebral bodies, or vertebra, provide the foundation and structure that allows us to be upright. The disc material is contained within the disc space by a tough, fibrous ring called the annulus fibrosus. The disc material in the center is gelatinous, made up mostly of water and proteoglycan (amino acids) termed the nucleus pulposus. Over time, the entire disc will lose integrity, much like a tire on a car. The outer ring of the disc, the annulus, can form a defect where disc material can extrude into the spinal canal.

There are many ways that a disc can herniate into the spinal canal. Disc herniations are among the most common causes of back and leg pain. It is also very common to find multiple disc herniations on an MRI at several different levels, and this does not necessarily correlate with the severity of a back condition. This is because disc herniations may or may not be contributing to your symptoms. In fact, as we read earlier in the introduction section, disc herniations can be observed on MRI in upwards of 50-60% of asymptomatic volunteers in their thirties!

## DISC HERNIATIONS CAN CAUSE PAIN BY COMPRESSION OF THE NEIGHBORING NERVE ROOT(S)

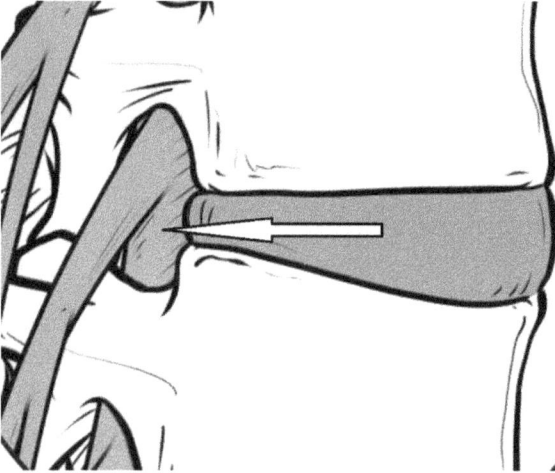

*The disc can put pressure on one or several nerves close coursing behind the disc space (arrow in figure). This can cause pain, and a number of other symptoms, such as numbness and weakness.*

## 24 What is the Difference Between a Disc Bulge, Protrusion, Extrusion, and Herniation?

A disc herniation comes in many forms, and for the most part, a radiologist who interprets an MRI will use these terms: bulge, protrusion, extrusion, and sequestration to describe the appearance of the disc herniation. Here are some of the terms and their definitions that you might find in your report, using the definitions from the American Society of Radiology as guidance:

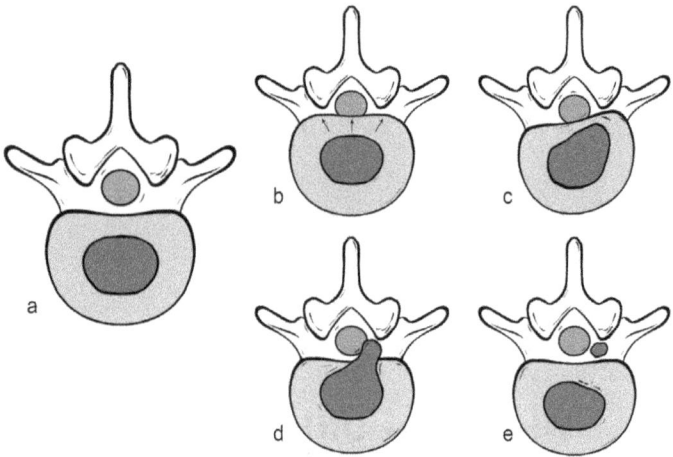

*Diagram depicting the various types of disc hernations. A. shows no her-niations. The spinal canal is depicted by red and is where the nerves are located. The disc space is in blue. B. A disc bulge is broad projection of the disc evenly outside of the disc space. C. A protrusion is where a small portion of the disc projects outside of the disc space, and less than 90 de-grees. D. A disc extrusion is where a fragment is outside of the disc space, and through the membrane surrounding the disc space. E. A sequestra-tion is a fragment of disc that is ouside of the disc space, not in continuity with the disc.*

## Types of Disc Herniations:

DISC BULGE

A disc bulge is where disc material projects beyond the margin of the vertebral body over more than 90 degrees of the circumference. Another way of conceptualizing this is that the base of the disc is equal to, or greater than half the disc diameter (example b in the diagram). These are the most common and occur in patients with and without symptoms. These frequently can cause symptoms on both sides, due to how concentric they are.

## PROTRUSION

Disc material projects beyond the vertebral body, but less than 90 degrees, and the base of projection is wider than the dome.

## EXTRUSION

Disc material has gone through a defect in the disc wall, in continuity with the disc space, often with the base narrower than the dome. Most often, extrusions cause symptoms, presumably as inflammatory material from the nucleus resides outside of the disc space to inflame an exiting spinal root.

## SEQUESTRATION

No direct continuity with the disc space. Disc material projects away from the disc space. This is the least commonly seen.

## 25 What is Stenosis and How Much is Too Much?

Stenosis is a narrowing of the diameter of any passage in the body. In the spine, stenosis is narrowing of the area where the nerve course through the spine. The spinal cord is comprised of nerves that run to and from the brain and is in the central canal of the spine. The nerves exit to the right and the left through a neural foramen. There are two main types of stenosis: foraminal stenosis, where single nerves are compressed as they exit the spine, and in the central canal where the nerves of the spinal cord can be compressed. In most people the spinal cord ends at the first lumbar segment and all of the lumbar and sacral nerves travel down the central canal, where they can be compressed in either the central canal or neural foramen.

Stenosis is very common. In an adult who is symptom

free without back or leg pain, there is just enough room for the nerves to run through the spine. Any kind of disc herniation, or arthritis of the spine, can cause a narrowing – and therefore can be described as stenosis by a radiologist (stenotic). This is a very common finding from an MRI.

Stenosis is occasionally graded as 'mild', 'moderate', and 'severe' and these qualitative terms differ. Just exactly what the variation 'moderately severe' means to the patient and what the clinical relevance is, remains to be seen. Qualitative grading of stenosis for a particular study may vary in interpretation, which is a common hurdle with some grading scales.

## 26   Do I Need Contrast With An MRI/CT?

Contrast (dye), refers to a chemical administered by the radiologist intravenously (for an MRI of the spine, contrast is given through the veins) with the sole purpose to increase the detection of certain diseases on spinal imaging. Scar tissue will also appear much more clearly after contrast is administered. Contrast is only helpful in specific disease processes, and most often, is not helpful for routine diagnostic imaging. The majority of clinical problems are degenerative spinal disorders and both CT and MRI imaging with contrast is not required. Also, these substances can be associated with severe allergic reactions and kidney failure among other conditions. For that reason, the risks outweighs the potential benefits of administering contrast during every imaging study.

## 27    What is Spondylolisthesis?

Spondylolisthesis is also known as the "slip" in the spine. This slip most commonly occurs at the disc space between the fourth and fifth lumbar vertebra. This condition develops as a result of degenerative disc disease. The disc degenerates and loses height, causing the suspensory ligaments to buckle (like jeans that are too long). The supporting forces that hold two levels together are gone and an abnormal sliding motion can occur horizontally at the disc between two vertebral levels. The body attempts to stabilize the spondylolisthesis by creating stabilizing forces, which it does by thickening the ligaments and joints. One consequence is that too much stenosis can develop centrally in the central canal or in the neural foramen where the nerve exits resulting in symptomatic nerve compression. This nerve compression is caused by the thickening of the ligaments, joint growth, and disc bulging.

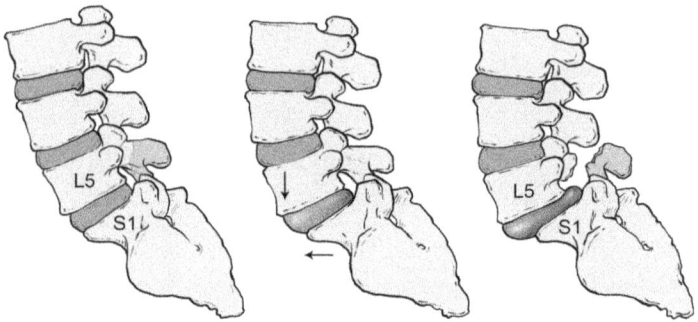

*Spondylolisthesis. Diagram above demonstrating the L5 vertebral body is prone to sliding in front of S1(center), due to the unique downward slope of the L5-S1 disc space(left). As the disc degenerates, the ligaments become less taut, and there is increased horizontal motion. This problem is even more common in those with steeper sloping discs. Eventually, this slip can progress further, and is associated with a fracture of the pars(spondylolysis) and disc herniations(right).*

Paradoxically, removal of these stabilizers is the treatment-nerve decompression. This can result in worsening spondylolisthesis and this forms the basis for the argument that fusion will be needed eventually for this problem. However, a decompression is appropriate as well, and certain clinical and imaging features may make you more likely to get a greater benefit from one type of surgery over another. Radiologists grade spondylolisthesis as Grades I, II, III, and IV, and is delineated by the extent of slippage: 0-25, 26-50, 51-74, and 75-100%.

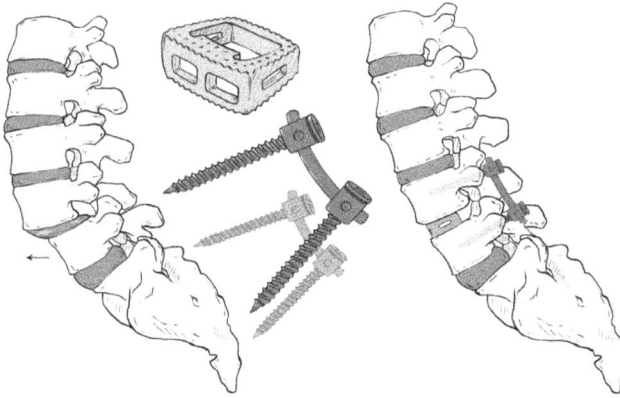

*Spondylolysis can cause debilitating back and leg pain from painful motion and nerve compression due to instability. The diagram above depicts the use of an interbody cage and pedicle screws to realign the spine and stabilize it. Over time, bone will grown across the level that was stabilized with screws, rods, and the cage.*

## 28  What is Spondylolysis (a.k.a. Pars Fracture, or Pars Defect)?

An important bridge of bone, called the pars interarticular (or pars), provides a degree of spinal stability by articulating with the adjacent facet joints above and below on the right and left side.  This is a thin bone that is subject to a high degree of stress, therefore subject to fracture. This is quite common, occuring often in adolescence.

Fracture of this bone is termed spondylolysis, which can be  a fracture on either the right or the left side, or often both sides. This is most common at the L5-S1 where biomechanical forces are greatest.  The term pars defect is used interchangeably with pars fracture, but has no unique significance. The pars provides biomechanical stability and prevents slippage, so a fracture may or may not be associated with spondylolisthesis (when associated, the term is spondylolisthesis *with* spondylolysis). Since there are other stabilizing structures, the degree of slippage is usually less than 25% (grade I). Having a pars fracture makes you susceptible to developing spondylolisthesis that may progress later on in life. These fractures do not heal on their own due to the poor blood supply. As a result, surgery is often required, which is a fusion.

## Key Points

- A spondylolysis, is a fracture of the pars that can cause back pain, leg pain, or both.
- Slippage of one verteba over the other can occur over time, resulting in low back pain and leg pain.
- This fracture generally doesn't heal without surgery.
- Bracing is not very effective.
- Spondylolysis most often requires surgery which results in back and leg pain relief.
- The surgical treatment is stabilization and fusion.
- A fusion relies on metal implants to immobilize two adjacent vertebra, wihch results in a loss of motion in the spine(decreased flexibility).

## 29    What Does Arthritis Look Like On a

## Spine Imaging Report?

There are many different confusing terms and they all represent the arthritis process. This is an age-dependent process. Just because they are there does not mean that they have to be removed immediately like a cancer.

| Common terms on my report | |
|---|---|
| Facet arthropathy | Inflammation in the facet joints, where there are two per level in the lumbar spine. These joints facilitate motion. |
| Spurs (osteophytes) | A sign of chronic 'wear and tear'. The body develops these bone spurs to distribute forces evenly through a disc level and to stabilize abnormal motion. |
| Degenerative disc | Loss of water and collagen in the disc, resulting in decreased space between the vetebra. |
| Modic changes | Describes inflammation in the bone adjacent to the degenerated disc (the endplate). |
| Ligamentous hypertrophy | Thickening of ligaments occur in response to abnormal motion at a particular level of the spine. |
| Stenosis | Narrowing of a space or channel, and in the spine this can cause compression of a nerve root. |

## 30   Do I Have Scoliosis?

Interestingly, discs can degenerate unevenly, which can cause changes in the weight-bearing forces on the spine, causing a cascade of uneven degeneration. This is a process known as degenerative scoliosis. To classify a patient as having scoliosis, many academic and professional surgeon societies have designated a minimal curvature of ten degrees to meet the criteria. Your report usually defines scoliosis as any curvature (1 degree or greater).

It is common for patients to think that they have scoliosis, but it is very frequent for adults to develop some spinal curvature from asymmetric disc degeneration. Uneven disc degeneration results in spinal curvature, because the rectangular disc becomes triangular in shape(image on right, figure below).

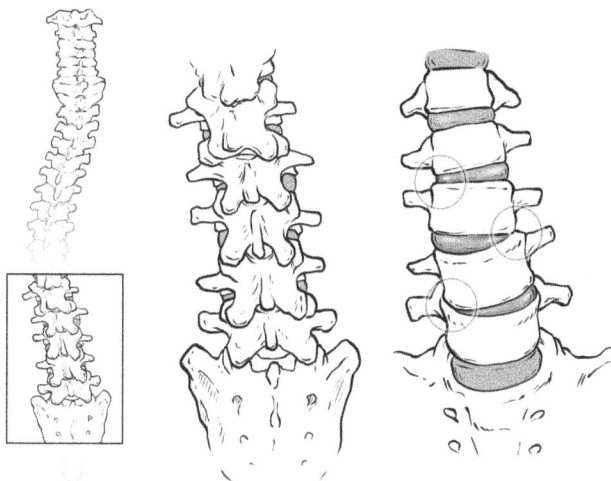

*Degenerative scoliosis. Examples of abnormal spinal curvature (diagram above) is most often due to uneven degeneration of the disc, resulting in uneven pressure across the disc space, and further increased degeneration. This can precipitate spinal curvation resulting in back pain and nerve compression.*

Not everyone with scoliosis need surgery. The surgical correction of scoliosis is a major surgical undertaking for most people. Spinal curvature, once it develops, leads to further loading of the spine unevenly. Arthritis once again accelerates as the bodies attempts to stabilize the spine and prevent the curvature from worsening. Once again, enlarged ligaments, joints, and disc herniations result in symptomatic stenosis. The stenosis can be anywhere across three general areas:

- Foraminal stenosis: Where the nerve exits.
- Central stenosis: The spinal canal, where the nerves travel after exiting and entering the spine.
- Lateral recess (subarticular) stenosis: narrowing underneath the facet joints. This occurs often where the curvature is greatest in the spine (at the apex of the curve).

When the patient becomes symptomatic from the scoliosis, they develop stenosis and compression of the exiting nerve in the neural foramen, or they develop narrowing of the central spinal canal and compression of the nerve or spinal canal that way. Decompression of the nerves in this situation, just like with spondylolisthesis, means to remove the stabilizing elements that took years to counterbalance the spine, resulting in destabilization. The way to prevent worsening scoliosis after decompression surgery is to place screws and rods to hold the spine in position after the decompression. Screws, rods, and other rigid mechanical implants such as cages that sit in between each spinal level are powerful tools to correct scoliosis and maintain a proper alignment. The exact indications for surgery to treat scoliois will require a separate book and there are patient specific factors to take into consideration- seek counsel from a spinal surgeon.

# What Are the Two most Common Types of Scoliosis?

| Type | Description |
|---|---|
| Degenerative (de novo) | Asymmetric age-related degeneration of the spine and disc resulting in curvature of the spine, where a curve exceeds 10 degrees. |
| Idiopathic scoliosis | A disorder where a segment of the spine is rotated, causing the spine to curve.<br><br>This is usually due to genetic causes. |

# SECTION IV

# NON-SURGICAL TREATMENT

# 31  Should I Take Medication?

Over the counter(OTC), non-steroidal anti-inflammatory drugs(NSAIDs),  are the preferred pain-relieving medications to be taken within the first month of acute low back pain.  With that said, while it is recommended early on within 1 month, the chronic use of NSAIDs carry an increased risks of side-effects.  Also, low-quality evidence has been published against the use of acetaminophen long term due to the minimum benefit.  It showed in one study a lack of difference compared to a placebo.  In general, the quality of medical studies are poor and they do not support the use of over-the-counter analgesics long term.

## Key Points

- Prescription analgesics are generally not recommended for acute low back pain, due to the risks outweighing the benefits.

- If you are in acute or chronic pain, then it is reasonable to explore all of your options with your physician or healthcare provider.

- Understand the risks of all medications that you take. The major NSAID side-effects involve but are not limited to the GI symptoms (from absorption of the medication), and elimination of the medication (kidney or liver).

- Avoid opiate use.

## What is the Difference Between Tylenol(acetaminophen) and Advil(ibuprofen)?

- Acetaminophen is primarily a pain-reliever, and not technically an NSAID, and has very little anti-inflammatory properties

- ibuprofen is an anti-inflammatory medication(NSAID)

- Of the over the counter medications, NSAIDs will be most helpful in relieving symptoms and they are driven by inflammation.

# Should I Use a Muscle Relaxant?

Muscle relaxers are one option that may help with pain control, particularly when youhave painful muscle spasms. Medical evidence shows that skeletal muscle relaxants improve short term pain when compared to placebo. Also, there is not much support for one muscle relaxer over another. Most muscle relaxants do not work primarily on the muscle cells themselves, but rather, they target the central nervous system, causing an intoxicating effect. They should not be used in conjunction with opiates as the perceived adverse effects are much greater.

## 32   What Should I Try During the First

## Month of Symptoms?

Below are a list of nonsurgical treatment therapies that can be effective within the first month of surgery. There are other options available. When choosing an option, it has to be right for you. These options below are excellent because they are shown to be helpful in alleviating low back pain. Since low back pain can often spontaneously improve, it is sometimes hard to know if low back pain improvement occurred due to the treatment, or if this was just going to happen anyway. As a result, if there are no red flag symptoms, it is adviseable to consider the therapies below, or generally any therapy that has a low risk profile, and is a non-invasive procedure.

| First Line Treatments |
|---|
| Physical Therapy |
| Stretching and Light exercise |
| Over the Counter Anti-inflammatory Drugs (NSAIDS) (eg acetaminophen, ibuprofen) |
| Chiropracter |
| Accupuncture |
| Massage |
| Dry Needling |
| Meditation |
| Yoga and Tai Chi |
| Meditation and Stress Reduction |
| Aquatherapy |
| Application of Heat or Ice |

## 33   Is it Safe For Me to Return to Work?

That all depends on the type of work that is being performed and the underlying cause of the pain. Healthcare providers have your health and safety as a number one concern. Each patient's situation is unique and You are unlikely to find a specific answer that suits your unique job description and medical history.

As a general rule, for most problems related to aging and degeneration of the spine without spinal cord or nerve compression causing weakness, there is insufficient scientific evidence that says it is unsafe to return to your job, or to limit activities of daily living. However, there are other factors that need to be considered when making this decision which can include other medical issues and surgeries, as well as specific occupational concerns. Therefore, you will need to absolutely see your primary care provider and have this discussion with them.

# Key Points

- The decision to return to work most likely will require an expert in spinal disorders (see your healthcare provider).

- Your physician or provider may not be comfortable determining your capacity to carry out specialized or specific tasks that they are not familar with. There are specialists who can assess specific limitations and provide a detailed summary, which is referred to as a functional capacity evaluation.

- Often, employers want to know what a person's percent disability is related to a medical issue. There are agreed upon, published formulas for determining this. Again, this is a service that not all healthcare providers routinely provide, and it has lifelong implications. Therefore, you will often have to find a healthcare provider who routinely provides this service, and this is not necessarily provided everywhere.

| Considerations before returning to work (consult your care provider or employer first): |
|---|
| • Use of opiates, controlled substances, or substances that impair concentration, *AND* |
| • Operation of a vehicle to commute, or during job. |
| • Operation of heavy machinery or dangerous equipment, or handling of dangerous materials. |
| • Safety to myself or other is potentially impacted. |

## 34   What Medication Should I Avoid Early On?

There is no specific rule about which medications should be avoided, just general guidelines.  However, be extremely cautious of the addictive potential of prescription pain relievers, and their negative effects. This cannot be overstated.

Drug overdoses are now the leading cause of death in the U.S. for people under age 55 (see *'Heroin addiction explained: How opioids Hijack the Brain*, NY Times Dec 18, 2018).

# How Can My Risk For Opiate Addiction be Assessed?

One helpful tool used by physicians to assess for addiction potential in the setting of chronic pain is the opiate risk tool (ORT). (A list of the opiates being prescribed and their relative strengths (effectiveness/potency) will be listed in the following section.)

## Opioid Risk Tool

| Opioid Risk Tool | | |
|---|---|---|
|  | Female | Male |
| Family history |  |  |
| Alcohol abuse | 1 | 3 |
| Prescription drug abuse | 2 | 3 |

| | | |
|---|---|---|
| Illicit drug use | 4 | 4 |
| Personal History | | |
| Alcohol abuse | 3 | 3 |
| Prescrip-tion drug abuse | 4 | 4 |
| Illicit drug use | 5 | 5 |
| Age 16-45? | 1 | 1 |
| History of preadoles-cent sexual abuse? | 3 | 0 |
| Psychiat-ric History? | 2 | 2 |
| Depres-sion | 1 | 1 |

Use the ORT above and use the table below to calculate the total score:

| Score | Risk |
|---|---|
| <4 | Low |
| 4-7 | Moderate risk |
| >7 | High |

## 35   Opiates Are a Last Resort

Opiate use is not considered a first-line therapy for short term pain. As mentioned before, this means that alternative medications should be considered beforehand. Opiates (eg. hydrocodone, oxycodone) quickly lose their effectiveness in treating pain, as the body quickly becomes tolerant to the dosage. Opiates should be careful considered under the direction of your healthcare provider.

# Key Points

- Opiates are a last resort medication.

- Avoid opiate prescriptions at all costs in the first three months, if possible.

- Opiates may be considered after all other analgesics have be attempts, including NSAIDs, muscle relaxers, and glucocorticoids, benzodiazepines. (see questions 8 and 31, for more information regarding medication alternatives)

## Brief List of Common Opiate Medications

| Medica-<br>tion<br>(drug name) | Common<br>Trade Name | Strength | Common-<br>ly available<br>with acet-<br>aminophen |
|---|---|---|---|
| Codeine | Tyle-<br>nol-Codeine<br>(No. 3/No. 4) | + | Yes |

| | | | |
|---|---|---|---|
| Hydroco-done | Vicodin/Norco (contains acetaminophen) | ++ | Yes |
| Oxyco-done | Oxycon-tin, Roxico-done | +++ | Yes (Trade name: Perco-cet contains tylenol) |
| Hydro-morphone | Dilaudid | ++++ | No |

## 36 **What Are the Dangers of Opiates?**

Opioids are now the leading cause of death under the age of 55. Death is due to a lack of adequate respiratory function, an effect of opiates. Often, combinations of prescription medications, or the use of alcohol while taking opiates cause increased side effects beyond what is expected. The following is a very brief summary highlighting only some of the most dangerous adverse effects of opiates, and a discussion of the risks of constipation, nausea, and urinary retention with opiates will more than likely occur in your PCP office:

## Addiction

These are highly addicting. Close to 10% of of those taking opioids develop temporary addictive behaviors or permanent addiction.

# Withdrawl

This can still be fatal, but far less severe relative to opiate overdose. Long term use increases the risk of withdrawl symptoms if opiate reduction isn't planned carefully.

# Tolerance

The body can become increasingly tolerant with prolonged use. There is no known maximum opiate dose, as the body can become tolerant to the side-effects with time.

# Respiratory Suppression

One of the most concerning effects is that decreased breathing occurs with higher doses, which can be fatal. It is estimated that 90 Americans die each day from an opioid overdose, and this is usually from respiratory arrest.

# Increased Sensitivity to Pain

This is the opposite of what you want opiates to do, and it happens, increasing your demand for more opiates. This is a component of what is seen with an increased tolerance, but what is really happening is the efficacy is steadily decreasing due to tolerance and an increased sensitivity to pain.

In other words, long term use of opiates at high doses may increase the likelihood of developing a hypersensitivity syndrome. More recent research suggests that the activation of glial cells(cells of your nervous tissue) increases interleukin-1 beta expression(inflammatory marker) which has been shown to increase chronic pain. The brain does increase the intensity of pain signals after prolonged opioid use partly out of an adaptation to be able to sense environmental threats.

## 37 What are Some of the Things I Can Do to Decrease My Low Back Pain Long Term?

There are numerous options for the treatment of low back pain.  For most people, low back pain will come and go, and it is a very common problem.  Additionally, for people with low back AND leg pain, this problem will also go away without any invasive treatments.  Below, I will list some common therapies that are considered beneficial for short term and long term low back pain reduction.  Advanced imaging, such as magnetic resonance imaging of the lumbar spine(MRI) is not recommended for most people with low back pain, without meeting strict criteria.  This is to help limit patients obtain unnecessary imaging studies, and to limit growing healthcare costs in North America.  There are two specific issues with obtaining an MRI too early after the onset of back pain:

- An MRI cannot link a specific 'finding'(a 'finding' is anything that the radiologist describes) with the cause of low back pain, since low back pain if vague, and not specific to the disc levels, the facet joints, or muscles and ligaments.

- An MRI does not sort out the difference between age-appropriate degeneration of the spine and disease.

# General Therapies Effective for Low Back Pain Reduction:

| |
|---|
| Weight loss (see question 38) |
| Core strengthening and physical therapy |
| Meditation |
| Stretching |
| Yoga |
| Massage |
| Aquatherapy |
| Tai Chi |
| TENS |
| Pharmacotherapy |
| Interventional Pain Management Techniques |

## 38 How Effective is Weight Loss?

Losing weight helps lower low back and leg pain. In one study showing a benefit of weight reduction in patients that underwent bariatric surgery, patients with LBP and/or leg pain were an average of 270 pounds before, and 176 lbs after surgery. Not only could it be shown that their low back and leg symptoms decreased, but the disc got taller! This 2 millimeter increase is substantial (25% increase) and occasionally often enough to take the pressure fully off of a nerve. Small changes in weight have not been well studied, and the biggest changes have been shown in patients with a BMI[3] over 35.

---

3    *The Body-mass index (BMI) is a ratio of your weight to height. This is calculated most commonly with the formula for the metric system: Weight (kg) / (Height in meters)². Normal is considered between 18.5 to 24.9, Overweight is considered 25-29.9, and obesity is regarded as 30 and over. A formula for using pounds and inches:  Weight (lbs) * 703 / (Height in inches)² .*

Losing weight at a time of severe low back pain is a difficult subject for patients. Often, it is mentioned that exercise
worsens the LBP, making weight loss an impractical way
to lower LBP. While the subject of weight loss in this book
will not go beyond this section, it is important to mention a
few things about losing weight. It is commonly taught that
1 pound of fat is 3500 calories. This number of calories is
an estimate and the range is roughly 2800-3700 calories. A
pound of body fat varies with regard to how much fat and
how much water, but there is roughly 454 grams of body fat
tissue in a pound, with 87% lipid (13% without caloric content - eg. water). which is 395 grams of lipids/fat per pound.
395 grams of lipids is multiplied by 9 calories per gram of
fat, and the total is 3555 calories per 1 pound of fat.

Your body has a daily caloric need, which simply
means the total daily calories you need to meet your demand - ie. without losing any weight. Lets use the general
example: 2500 calories in a day. For all practical purposes,
losing weight requires a strict knowledge of your daily calorie intake by keeping a log of everything you eat and drink.
So, the bottom line is, eat less calories than you require, an
every 3500 calories below your needs, you lose 1 pound of
body fat.

It is helpful to be as consistent as possible from day to
day. For somone who needs 2500 calories per day, if they
ate 2000 calories per day, after 7 days, they are 3500 calories
below their requirement, and they would reach a target of 1
lb per week. If you were to take a day or two off from your
diet, or miss dessert in your log, the daily 500 calorie deficit
may not be reached. It is easy to then realize how hard it is
to diet because of the consistency required.

Also, as you lose weight, your metabolism will decrease
due to weight loss and a general mechanism to prevent star-
vation, and as a result your daily calorie needs will decrease.

This leads to a lack of results after some early weight loss, which can be discouraging and lead to abandoing a diet. However, Your daily needs change as your weight changes.

What are other ways to lose weight? You can have a calorie deficit by exercise, or limiting either your appetite or metabolism by medication. These are important to know since exercise is often too painful with LBP problems. Medications and surgery can specifically be helpful to lose weight, and require a consultation with a bariatric medicine specialist. A nutritionist is likely an expert you should work with beforehand to make sure you have worked hard on optimizing your diet, which can lead to results, without the risks of medication and surgery.

## 39 How Does Physical Therapy, Core Strengthening, and Other Conditioning Activities help?

There are numerous examples of patients that have been helped with physical therapy in the setting of acute LBP. The most straightforward answer is that most acute LBP will resolve spontanteously without treatment.  It is hard to then show physical therapy alters the natural history of something if the desired outcome happens regardless. However, it goes beyond that explanation.  Strength-training, targeted physical training, and core muscle conditioning have been shown in numerous studies to effectively help patients avoid more expensive and invasive low back pain treatments.

In the most general terms, physical therapy for low back pain can be grouped into three broad categories of exercises that each can help you with low back pain and be preventative against future episodes:

# Stretching

Helps maintain normal range of motion, provide relief for muscles in spasm due to abnormal posture, and muscle spasms from painful nerve irritation.

# Dynamic Stabilization Exercises

Dynamic stabilization entails exercises that rely heavily upon stabilizing muscle through various ranges of motion. One example of this would be using exercise balls, which require stabilizing core muscles to keep you balanced on the exercise ball.

# Core Strengthening Exercises

Traditional exercises that increase muscle bulk through the abdominal muscle group and posterior spinal muscles. One example of core-strengthening would be weighted-machine crunches and hyperextensions.

# Key Points

- Prior to beginning a new exercise program, always discuss your plans with a healthcare professional.

- There are numerous physical therapy exercises, and further detail is beyond the scope of this book. I would recommend at the very least, a consultation with a physical therapist to obtain a professional evaluation and to develop a training program with goals in mind. This will help avoid injury maximize your chances of successfully completing your planned therapy.

- Keep this in mind, patients that complete a physical therapy program are less likely to seek out more invasive low back pain treatments.

- Having chronic back problems should not be regarded as a reason to avoid physical therapy. If you are concerned with injuring yourself during physical therpay, then a physical therapist can guide you safely through the process.

- Some chronic medical conditions, obesity/morbid obesity, and a lack of physical conditioning makes physical therapy challenging for some people. Physical therapists and their teams strive to help patients with these hurdles.

## 40   What is an Epidural Steroid

## Injection?

An epidural steroid injection(ESI) decreases nerve inflammation in a more precise manner by allowing a concentrated delivery of steroids to the area immediately around
the inflammed nerve. Steroids provide long activing pain
relief for either leg or low back back pain. Inflammation of
the nerves is a common cause of this back pain and pain
shooting down your leg(radicular pain). This procedure is
performed in an office setting under minimal sedation and
local anesthesia (the skin is temporarily made numb with
an injection).  You will be awake for this procedure, but
with medication to help limit your discomfort. Often the
pain relief is very helpful, and can help you avoid surgery.
Epidural steroid injections are considered to be the most

effective non-surgical treatment of LBP or leg pain.

## Selective Nerve Root Block

A selective nerve root block is when the physician injects an anesthetic only (for example, lidocaine), which temporarily blocks nerve transmission, shutting off pain, and all sensation as well as motor function supplied by that nerve. This is useful in certain instances when it is unclear of the cause of pain.

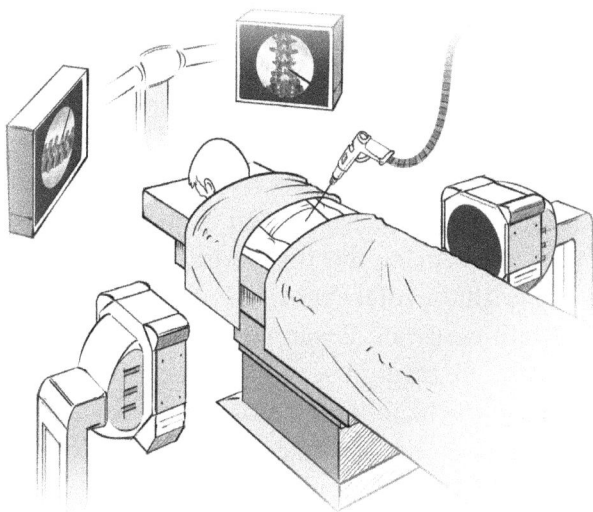

*Diagram showing layout of procedure room. The patient is undergoing spinal injection(surgeon removed from illustration). You are laying flat on a special table, and your back is sterily cleaned. X-rays are used to guide a needle to the appropriate region of the spine, and the pain doctor use the xrays to guide the needle.*

# What is a Transforaminal Epidural Steroid Injection?

A transforaminal epidural steroid injection guides steroids precisely to the area surrounding the nerve and epidural space(area around the spinal canal with the nerves and spinal cord) at the region of the neural foramen – the bony channel where each nerve root exits the spine. For each procedure, x-rays are used to guide the needle to localize the appropriate level and also to avoid needle injury to the nerve root. Using x-ray and a special dye that blocks x-ray from passing through(contrast), the pain management doctor can confirm that the needle is in the appropriate space around the nerves, and then use the contrast to confirm with x-rays that the steroid and sometimes other analgesics are injected around the nerves. Ionizing radiation is used during this procedure, which is a risk for cancer, although the total exposure is minimal.

Some facilities use a CT scanner to provide very precise injections, but the amount of radiation exposure is significantly greater. The benefits of a more sophisticated imaging system over a fluoroscopic image has not been demonstrated in studies. Epidural steroid injections are helpful for pain caused by disc herniations and foraminal stenosis. Some studies show that patients can improve up to 6 weeks after an ESI.

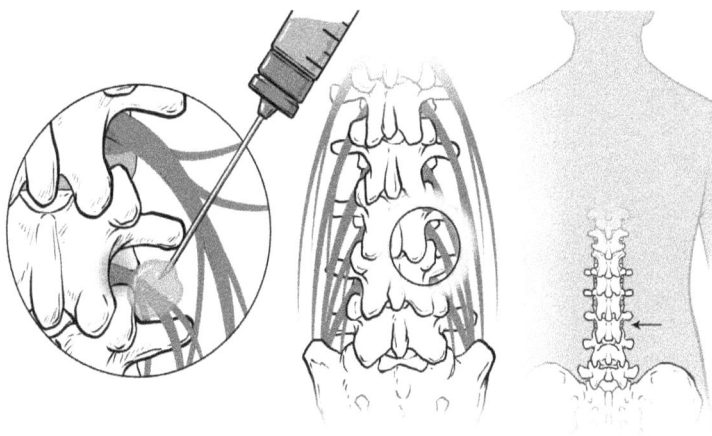

*of your low back in relation to your spine. (center image) The nerves can be targetted as they exit the spine, as shown in the diagram. This is thought to be more selective, since medication will be concentrated on the symptomatic nerve root. (figure left) Transforaminal Injections target specifically one exiting nerve at the level of the foramen.*

## What if I Don't Get Better From an Injection, Should I Try Another?

Less than 10% of patients may benefit from a second injection. If a second injection can be obtained within a reasonable time period and you can hold off from seeking a surgeon, then it would be adviseable to see if a second injection is a benefit. This decision is based on your specific case, and a discussion with the physician who is performing your injections will help you decide this.

# 41 What is a Lumbar Facet Injection?

There is a right and left facet joint that connects each level of your back. This joint can cause back pain. A lumbar facet (zygoapophyseal) intraarticular joint injection delivers steroids to the pair of joints between each vertebra in the spine. Lumbar facet pain ranges from 15 to 60% of LBP, according to previously published studies. Facet joints are covered with these nerve fibers that carry mainly pain sensation and very little else.

# Key Points

- Lumbar Facet Injections are an effective treatments for low back pain.

- These injections often provide relief, lasting months.

- The procedure is similar to an epidural steroid injection (*see chapter 40, epidural steroid injection*), except the target is the facet joint.

- These procedures are most often followed by a radiofrequency ablation.

- Further injections are often needed in the future for maintenance of pain relief.

## 42   What is Radiofrequency Ablation?

Radiofrequency ablation(RFA) is a very effective treatment of low back pain, when back pain is felt to be caused predominantly by the small joints in the back, called the facet joints. An RFA is performed by a pain management physician, in the office or hospital setting. The procedure begins with a local anesthetic to block pain fibers from  different joints in the back. If a significant portion of pain is reduced by blocking a facet joint, then the  medial branch nerves can be burned(ablated) using radio waves. This is an excellent treatment for low back pain that has a high likelihood of being effective at a 1 and 2 year follow-up.

# Key Points

- Lumbar facet joint pain is a recognized cause of chronic back pain.

- Facet joint blocks using local anesthetics are performed in the clinic by pain management physicians. The blocks help identify the joints contributing to low back pain.

- Medial branch nerves are nerve fibers found on the surface of the facet joints, which can be  burned in a process to decrease pain signals, in a process called radiofrequency ablation (RFA).

- RFA uses radiofrequency waves to generate heat, which in turn damages the nerve endings.

- This procedure has been shown to be very effective in decreasing back pain, when the lumbar facet joints are identified as a main contributor of back pain.

# SURGICAL TREATMENT

# 43    How Do I Know if I Need Surgery?

The short answer is that you will be unable to know for sure without a consultation from a spinal surgeon, and the advice of your primary care provider. The practice of medicine requires years of education and training to develop these skills required to answer questions like these. The more you can learn about your spinal condition and your options, the better off you will be, because you can make the most well-informed decision.

In the persuit of becoming more informed through the internet, it is now very common to be exposed to personal reviews for just about anything offered in healthcare. These reviews are helpful as they educate us as patients to ask the best possible questions and to better understand a surgical procedure. However, a surgeon will not be able to explain why someone had a particularly good or bad experience, or why another patient had one type of surgery or not. Risk varies from patient to patient, and in order to maintain strict healthcare confidentiality, patient information will not be shared, ever.

Aside from that, while your risk of a complication varies depending on the type of operation you have, their are so many variables that come into play, it is beyond the scope of this discussion. Your surgical risk (complications), can be grouped into things that raise your risk (your medical, surgical, and social history), the planned operation (complexity of the surgery), and the postoperative period. A discussion with your surgeon should include a discussion of risk, as it will help you understand the nature of the surgery better.

# Key Points

- Most people will not need surgery

- Most people that require surgery for a degenerative condition of the spine should attempt to exhaust all nonsurgical measures before considering surgery.

- The right surgeon for you is someone you trust, has thoroughly explained your condition to you and your treatment options, and has discussed surgery with you including appropriate expectations and whether or not the goals of surgery and the surgeons expecations are in line with yours.

## 44  What Are the Roles of A Spine

## Surgeon?

The traditional role of a spinal surgeon has always been as a surgical consultant, who sees patients who were referred after a careful consideration that the spinal problem requires surgery as the principle means to getting better. A spinal surgeon has expertise in treating disorders of the spine surgically after careful consideration of appropriate nonsurgical management. In the majority of situations with early onset low back pain and leg pain, surgical intervention is not warranted. Therefore, a spinal surgery evaluation is not required up front.

With that said, the role has shifted over time for many spinal surgeons. Some surgeons provide many nonsurgical treatments and therefore are comfortable seeing patients without having had prior nonsurgical therapies such as physical therapy and epidural steroid injections.

## 45 What is Minimally-Invasive Spine

## Surgery?

Minimally invasive spine surgery(MISS) is a very general term that describes the process of how the spine is exposed by the surgeon. Until more recently, spinal surgery has had the reputation of being a painful type of surgery, with a long and painful recovery. Although this depends on a number of factors, such as the purpose of the surgery, number of levels, and whether there was prior spinal surgery, the traditional approach to the spine('midline approach') has typically involved a vertical incision in the middle of the back, where the muscles and soft tissues are split, and removed from the surface of the bone, where the muscles insert.

With the traditional approach, prolonged retraction under pressure is often required for the surgeon to have adequate view of the nerves and anatomy of the spine. At the end of the surgery, the muscle tension is released, but some of the muscle tissue will necrose(muscle cells will die, and atrophy) causing pain. The muscular attachments cannot be reattached to the bone, and in many cases, most of the bone where the muscles attached do not have any bone to reattach to, because they were removed to accomplish the operation. With traditional surgery, this creates an area where fluid can accumulate, and increases the risk of spinal infection.

Minimally-invasive approaches use dilators to make an opening in the muscle where a tube the diameter of approximately two cm is used to approach the spine. Small windows are made in the bone with very minimal removal of muscle from the point of insertion. Large retractors that cause prolonged muscle pain are not used with MISS. As a result of dilating the muscle, the muscle falls back into position when the tube is removed, and there is no cavity where fluid collects(no drain is needed), lowering the risk of infection.

Surgeons debate the exact definition, and some medical societies have defined MISS. If fusion surgery is planned for you, minimally-invasive surgery might be helpful for you. In select patients, minimally-invasive alternatives are becoming available for many procedures. Often minimally-invasive surgery may not be an option for you and at the time of this writing, there are not MISS alternatives for every surgical problem.

## POSTERIOR LUMBAR MINIMALLY-INVASIVE APPROACH

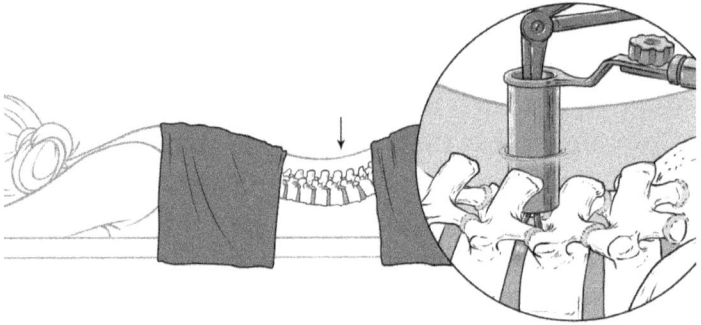

*Minimally invasive surgery involves dilators that expand the muscle, rather than removing them from the point where they insert into the bone. For the most part, this results in less postoperative pain, and less wound healing complications. Since less of the spine is seen during surgery, x-rays are taken in the operating room to visualize the spine.*

## 46  What is Laser Spine Surgery?

Laser spine surgery refers to the placement of a laser in the center of a disc, which in turn creates heat that burns the center of a disc, and possibly shrinking the disc and re-lieving nerve root compression. This uses a low level laser (acronym for the laser is Ho:YAG) and one general medical term for this is a nucleoplasty. A nucleoplasty was a popu-lar therapy used previously using where chemicals such as chymopapain, an enzyme, would be injected into the center of the disc to dissolve the nucleus. The end result is the de-crease in the total disc pressure(intradiscal pressure).

The decreased disc pressures result in the overall de-crease in the pressure of the disc thought to be the main inciter causing symptomatic nerve compression and leg pain. This can be accomplished through a channel created by a needle and a small dilator.  There are certainly patients that have felt symptomatic relief from this procedure, but a summary of the medical studies shows mixed results.

At the present time, you will not find many people offer-ing laser spine surgery for any type of degenerative spinal disorder because of the lack of long term benefit.

# 47 What is a Discectomy?

A discectomy is the removal of disc material. When that disc material is compressing a nerve, the a discectomy might be performed, which is a removal of the portion of herniated disc that is compressing the nerve. When an interbody fusion is being performed, a discectomy refers to removal the entire disc.

If a fusion is not performed, removal of the entire disc would result in pain and instability. The disc space serves a function and removing the entire disc is not typically performed without a fusion. The process of a discectomy can be performed either 'Open' or in a minimally-invasive fashion. With a minimally-invasive discectomy, a dilator is used to split the muscles overlying the lumbar spine, to approach the disc space. Some surgeons do not use the minimally-invasive approach, as the difference in incision between open and minimally-invasive spine (MIS) approaches is so small that in the case of a one-level discectomy, the difference in postoperative pain is often not substantial. As mentioned in the section about MIS, there are unique considerations that make MIS surgey more technically challenging to the surgeon, and may not be ideal for everyone.

## 48 **What is a Laminectomy?**

A laminectomy is a spinal procedure where the bone covering the back of your spinal canal is removed in order to relieve symptoms of nerve compression. This is the most common surgery to treat stenosis. Stenosis refers to a narrowing of a channel in the body. Most often people have heard about stenosis of arteries in the body, which causes symptoms by restricting blood flow.

Depending on the severity of your nerve compression, not only is the lamina removed from the center of the spine, along with the underlying ligaments, but some of the right and left facet joint as well. This procedure is commonly done in a same day surgery, but for some patients, a laminectomy performed over several levels may require an overnight stay in the hospital, or longer. In general, recovery from this procedure is relatively quick.

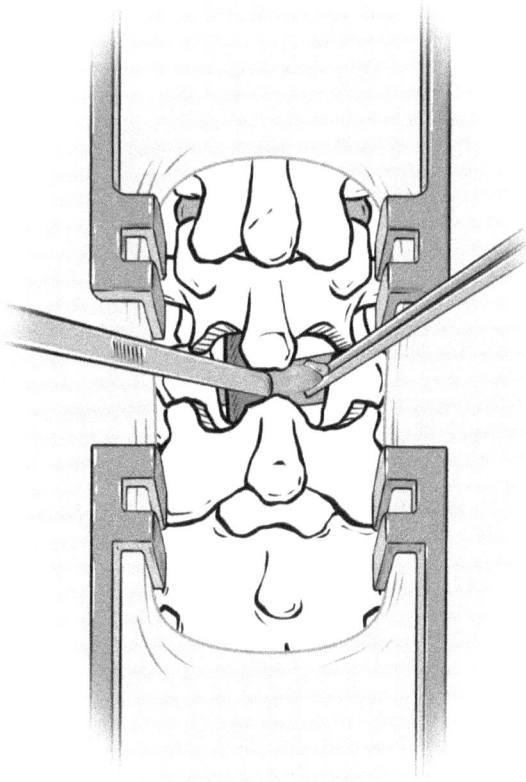

*Diagram depicting the removal of a disc herniation. Typically the incision allows the surgeon to see only the level of interest where the discectomy is being performed. In this diagram, a laminectomy is performed (bone removed covering the canal), and the nerve retracted to the left, while a tool removes the herniated disc.*

## 49 What is a Spinal Fusion?

Spinal fusion surgery is a surgical procedure where hard-ware is placed in the spine with the goal to facilitate the growth of bone across (fusing) a segment of the spine. The goal of a fusion is to remove motion entirely across a joint. This 'segment' that the bone grows across is a region where motion normally has occured.

## Indications

There are several indications for fusion surgery. Often, in the lumbar spine, this can be used for spondylolisthesis, disc herniations that recur after a prior discectomy, scoliosis, and spondylolisthesis due to pars fractures (spondylolysis). There are many more indications for fusion surgery and these can be thought of as any situation where there is abnormal and painful motion in the spine, or where enough bone will be resected that abnormal and painful motion may occur after the procedure is performed. One good example of this is seen in scoliosis due to degenerative disc disease. In this type of scoliosis, the disc degenerates on one side first, causing uneven loading of your body weight onto the side of the disc collapse, resulting in degeneration of multiple discs, all on the same side, resulting in a a spinal curvature (scoliosis). The ligaments and facet joints respond to the stresses of this abnormal curvature causing growth of the joints and thickening of the ligaments, which in turn can compress nerves. As you can see, if you were to remove the joints and ligaments to relieve painful nerve compression, the pain might be relieved temporarily, but the spinal curvature will increase resulting in worse scoliosis and more severe nerve root compression. The treatment then is a decompression followed by a fusion.

## Instrumentation and Fusion

Bone will best grow across a motion segment of the spine with a scaffold of bone that the surgeon places across the segment that is being fused. Surgeons often use donor bone (processed and treated bone from a cadaver) because there is not enough bone from your own spine to lay across the motion segment.

## Fusion and Nonfusion

The rates of fusion have improved over time with improvements in the hardware that provide more rigid fixation of the spine, and the guidance systems that allow for precision placement of the hardware. The fixation hardware will not withstand the stresses of your body forever. It was quickly realized that bone is more likely to grow across an area of motion, if it is stabilized with implants that connect the area above and below the region of motion. If your bone does not fully grow across this area of motion, the daily stresses on these implants could lead to loosening of the implants, cage or screw migration with painful nerve compression, or rod and screw breakage.

## How New Technology Might Impact Fusion

The evolution of implants has been a process of improving implant design to achieve the following desirable characteristics: increased durability, increased stability, and increased safety of placing the implants into the spine. Many factors affect the likelihood of bone fully bridging across an area of motion. Fusion can occur anytime within three to twelve months.

Often, bone removed to decompress the nerves is saved and used for the fusion mass. Also, this bone is frequently not enough, and donated bone (allograft) is also placed in the fusion site. There are many alternative products to facilitate the fusion, including proteins and cells that are thought to stimulate fusion and synthetic bone which is rich in calcium and minerals thought to support the fusion.

An in-depth discussion of fusion techniques and considerations such as implants and fusion supplements are well-beyond the scope of this book. However, understanding specific risk factors for not having a fusion(called pseudoarthrosis) such as tobacco use, is an important discussion to have with your physician.

## STABILIZATION OF SPONDYLOLISTHESIS WITH PEDICLE

## SCREWS, RODS, AND AN INTERBODY CAGE

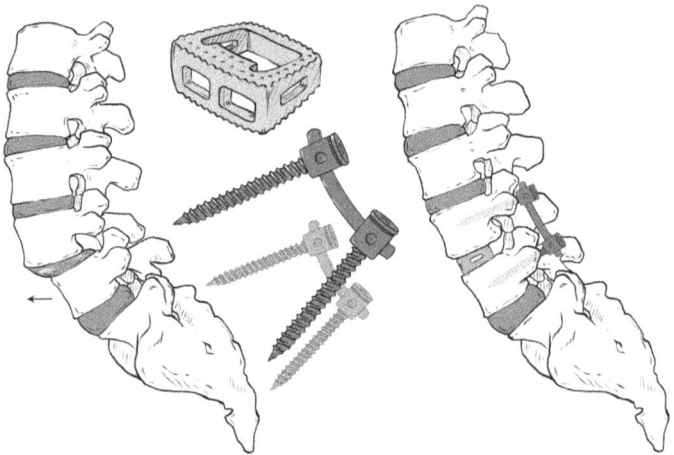

*Diagram depicting Lumbar 4-5 interbody fusion(spine on right) using a plastic polymer cage and titanium pedicle screws and rods(center) for stabilization of a spondylolisthesis(left). One way the cage stabilizes the spine is that it counteracts the horizontal(see arrow in the left figure) forces of the spine and increases stability.*

# Key Points

- Fusion(arthrodesis) consists of two time frames: a surgical component and the process of fusion, where bone bridges across an immobilized region of the spine.

- In fusion surgery, a surgeon immobilizes a region of the spine with screws and rods, a plate, or some other implant that results in no movement across a previously mobile area. The screws and rods are typically are not removed.

- Over the next 3 -12 months, bone cells slowly grow across this fusion bridge and bone is deposited.

- While a fusion results in less range of motion, the overall goal is to restore your quality of life.

## 50   What Are Some of the Most Common

## Risks of Surgery?

Every surgery has a risk of a complication.  Since each patient has a unique medical and surgical history, this discussion is best left to a detailed discussion that you should have
with your surgeon.

It is important for you to understand that the term risk
and the term 'complication' can have a variable meaning.
Instead, ask yourself what your expectations of surgery are,
and see if the surgeon has the same expecations as you do.
Then determine what are the things that can happen in surgery, and after surgery.  Then, see if there is any long term

risks. Long term risks from a fusion could involve a failure to fuse, possibly rod breakage, or symptomatic narrowing at the adjacent level of the spine, or even persistent pain without improvement.

## General Complication Categories: Preoperative, Intraoperative, and Postoperative

One helpful way to group complications in your mind, and to assist you in asking the most helpful questions is to think of the complications that can occur. When it comes to degenerative disc diseases that require surgery, there are relatively less preoperative complications to consider. One way to help you conceptualize these general groups is to use the example of a patien that needs a lumbar discectomy, but uses a blood thinner to prevent blood clots. The patients doctor tells them that stopping coumadin carries the risk of forming other blood clots. So, a requirement of most spinal surgeries by most spinal surgeons is to stop blood thinners several days before surgery. This is to make the surgery safe and prevent major bleeding. The preoperative complication risks come from stopping the blood thinner. The likelihood of having this problem varies, depending on the reason for needing blood thinners. In surgery, abnormal bleeding may still occur, depending on the blood thinner. Major blood loss would be an intraoperative risk. Postoperatively, restarting the blood thinner is necessary due to the blood clot risk. There is no guidance as to exactly how soon it can safely be started after surgery. If it is started too soon, the risks are developing a large collection of blood in the wound itself(hematoma) and possibly severe pain or a neurological problem from compression of nerves by the hematoma.

This would be an example of the postoperative risk. Not all examples of risk and complications occur before, during, and after surgery, like the example of blood thinner use. Howevere, this is a great example to illustrates how your unique medical issues impact your chances of having a complication, and this can occur at any time before, during, or after surgery.

# General Examples of Surgical and Medical Risks of Spinal Surgery[4]:

•Infection

•Persistent or worsening pain, or limited duration of pain relief

• A need for further spinal surgery

•Blood loss requiring a transfusion

•Pneumonia

•Blood clots (deep venous thrombosis, or DVT)

•Failure of fusion

•Accelerated degeneration at the normal disc below or above a fusion at the adjacent segment (called adjacent segment disease)

---

4     *This is a brief list and a consultation with healthcare profession is required for a detailed discussion of the risks and benefits of any medical therapy. A recurring theme throughout this book is that many medical details that are specific to you influence your likelihood of having a particular desired or undesired outcome.*

## 51    Will I Need More Lumbar Spine

## Surgery in the Future?

It is important to know that if you are having your first spinal surgery, there is a chance that you can require a more spinal surgery. Whether or not you need spinal surgery in the future depends on risk factors unique to your medical health, your lifestyle(eg. tobacco use), and the type of spinal surgery being performed. The technology of spinal surgery is not perfect and we are operating on mobile machinery designed for lifetime use.

If you have a discectomy, the entire disc is not removed, but a piece that has come out of a tear in the annulus(which makes a natural lining that surrounds the disc space). This tear cannot be repaired(although an interbody fusion in-volves removal of the whole disc and a cage is placed in the disc space to promote fusion). There is a a risk of a re-her-

niation which is thought to be due to the defect in the lining. In one study of patients who had a prior discectomy, 12
percent of patients underwent reoperation over four years,
and 6% underwent lumbar fusion.

More complex surgeries increase the risk of a need for
more spinal surgery. When a fusion is performed, a segment
of the spine that was previously flexible becomes more stiff,
and exerts more force on the levels above and below. The
longer the fusion segment, the more force that is exerted
on the level above or below. Up to 25% of people who have
lumbar spinal fusion procedure may become symptomatic
at adjacent levels within 10 years of their fusion operation.

## 52 Can a Lumbar Disc Be Replaced?

Lumbar disc replacement is not currently offered in the United States. Lumbar disc replacement therapy was offered for a short time. The appeal to this surgery was that it would allow for decompression of the nerves to the extent that fusion surgery provides, and simultaneously allow for motion at that level of surgery.

When it was offered, the surgery involved an incision in the abdomen, where the entire disc could be accessed and replaced by a large mechanical joint, the same concept with modern joint replacement procedures. Unfortunately, artificial discs in the lumbar spine had biomechanical issues resulting in debilitating back pain. Ultimately, these artificial discs were no longer offered due to the high number of complications associated with it. At the present time, spinal surgeons in the United States do not offer lumbar disc replacement procedures.

## 53   Do I Need Surgery For a 'Disc'?

One common theme in this book and in medicine in general, is that general medical advice does not necessarily apply to everyone.  This also applies to degenerative disc disease, which includes disc herniations.  How common is a disc herniation, disc bulge, disc extrusion, disc protrusion, degenerative disc, and/or disc sequestration?  It is so common that odds are that if a 40 year old without symptoms were to  get a lumbar spine MRI today, they are more likely than not to have one of these findings identified by the radiologist, including the diagnosis of degenerative disc disease.  Therefore, it is unlikely to draw the conclusion that surgery is possibly needed, just by having one of those above-mentioned findings.

When pain is the only symptom, and the problem is thought to be a large disc herniation, it is best to attempt all available nonsurgical therapies that are within your means.  Most disc herniations will improve on there own, and surgery is not required in 3 months. Physical therapy is a common initial recommendation for back pain. However, most people do not have a budget that accomodates for an extra 80 dollars, several times a week. But there are numerous other nonsurgical therapies. When it comes to treatments for a degenerative disease, especially disc herniations, surgery is the last resort.

Surgery carries risks, and no matter how rare a certain complication might be, if it happens to you, then it could be a life threatening problem. Surgery for disc herniations best help when the symptom is leg pain. Sometimes, in the case of a very large disc herniation, severe spinal stenosis can result causing both leg pain and back pain, causing difficulty walking and standing straight (symptoms of leg pain referred to as 'neurogenic claudication').

Despite your best efforts at avoiding surgery, sometimes it becomes necessary. Additionally, one helpful question to ask yourself is if you cannot complete the basic daily activities that are essential to you. However, the best way to make that determination is at the recommendation of your surgeon.

## 54   Does Spinal Surgery Improve Low

## Back Pain?

Low back pain improvement after surgery is no guarantee. Results vary and that highlights the importance with seeing a specialist in spinal disorders for a workup. To make another generalization, spinal surgery is more likely to result in a greater improvement in leg pain versus low back pain.

There are many conditions that cause LBP and your LBP may be caused by a number of things. For example, low back pain could be due to inflammation arising from disc spaces and the neighboring tissues across multiple spinal levels.  Examples of pain generators also include the facet joints and discs (discogenic pain), and/or painful muscular and ligamentous strain, or even sacroiliac (SI Joint) joint pain. There are many more causes (see section 1).  Often, leg pain due to a pinched nerve (radiculopathy) is more predictable and more reliably would improve with surgery.

Fundamentally, the surgery itself creates an entirely separate type of back pain, and back pain that heals slowly in the case of fusion surgery. Consider this likely scenario: You have back pain and you get an MRI. The MRI shows L2-3, L3-4, L4-5, and L4-5 findings: Four levels have varying degrees of "degeneration". Two discs are bulging, one is protruded, and one has severe degeneration where this is no disc left. Which level is causing the back pain? At one level, there is such severe degeneration tha there is almost no disc left, but could it be causing the specific pain that I have? As we mentioned, there are many drivers of low back pain, and this is what makes the process very difficult.

## 55   When Should I Consider Spinal Cord Stimulation?

Spinal cord stimulation is an FDA-approved surgical treatment for both back and leg pain provided by some surgeons- usually performed by spinal surgeons and pain management doctors.

A small, rechargeable battery and generator are implanted underneath the skin where electrical impulses are carried by wires that are tunnelled to the spinal cord. The wires stimulate part of the spinal cord that normally carries pain messages travelling up to the brain. The result is a decreased overall pain signal and often patients describe an increased tingling sensation. The circuitry of the spinal cord is very complicated, and the results vary per patient. As a result, a temporary spinal cord stimulator is placed prior to undergoing the surgery, and the results are observed.

If you experience a consistent pain reduction of greater than 50%, then surgeons will consider moving forward with a spinal cord stimulator.

At the present time, a battery that provides the electrical stimulation has a limited duration before it has to be replaced, in a surgical operation under general anesthesia. Howevere, rechargeable batteries are entering the market, which recharge using wireless induction which is becoming increasingly more common with  new cell phones. This may eventually allow most people to avoid operations to change the generator battery.

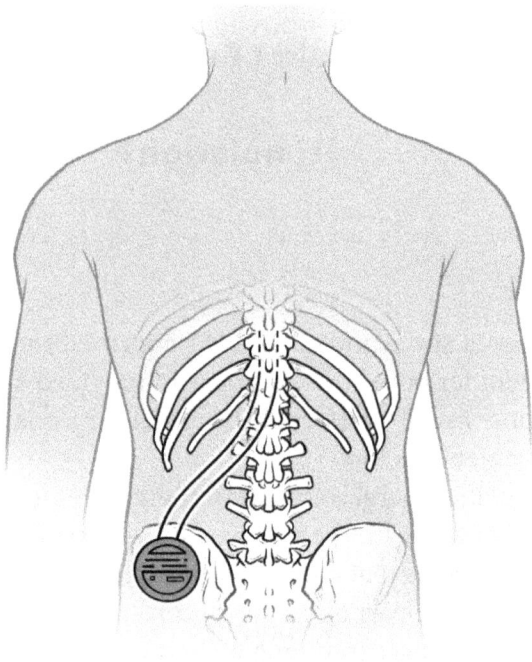

*Diagram depicting the spinal cord stimulator. A battery-generator pocket is placed above the hip, wires are tunnelled into the space, and stimulator leads rest just above the spinal cord. The intended effect is to decrease both back and leg pain signals.*

# 56  Are Stem Cell Injections Into The Disc

# a Safe and Helpful Way to Treat Low Back

# Pain?

At the present time, the injection of stem cells or cellular replacement therapy(cells other than 'stem cells') into the disc
is not established as an effective therapy. This treatment is
not FDA-approved and as more and more centers offer this
treatment, it is not FDA approved and potentially harmful.

However, several FDA approved trials are currently un-
derway. In these trials, cells are utilized for injections into
the disc space. These cells are thought to be ideal as they
can release anti-inflammatory chemicals into the disc space,
an area of inflammation. It is also hoped that cellular injections may be designed in the future to regenerate the disc
material and help prevent the natural process of degenerative disc disease. Although these studies began years ago,
it will be a long time before they reach the market, should
they ever be demonstrated to be helpful.

## Helpful Resources

There are numerous books and internet resources. The two books below are examples of straightforward, helpful books from physicians. Ultimately, when it comes to educational material and internet resources, there is a point where if major medical decisions have to be made, it is suggested that these major medical decisions be made under the guidance of a trusted physcian or healthcare expert.

I'll end and begin this book with a car analogy. If this book were about rebuilding brakes or a steering column on a classic car, one would hope that after your first rebuild of the breaks and/or steering column, you wouldn't go straight to the track without showing what you have learned to an expert, before potentially placing yourself in harms way.

BOOKS

- Back Pain by Loren Fishman, M.D., and Carol Ardman

- The End of Back Pain, by Patrick A. Roth, M.D.

INTERNET RESOURCES

- Spinalconfusion.wordpress.com: A blog written by a spinal surgeon. Provides clear and easily understandable descriptions of diseases, surgeries, and other treatments.

- www.spineuniverse.com: A great tool for patients and healthcare providers regarding the lastest treatment options, as well as education about the spine, common spinal problems, and all of the surgical and non-surgical treatment options.

- www.spine.org/knowyourback: This is a great spinal education resource and is provided by the North American Spine Society, which is a large multidisciplinary medical organization focusing on education, research, and both evidence and value-based spinal care.

# References

1.Bressler HB, Keyes WJ, Rochon PA, Badley E. The prevalence of low back pain in the elderly. A systematic review of the literature. *Spine (Phila Pa 1976).* 1999;24(17):1813-1819.

2.Pengel LH, Herbert RD, Maher CG, Refshauge KM. Acute low back pain: systematic review of its prognosis. *BMJ.* 2003;327(7410):323.

3.Docking RE, Fleming J, Brayne C, et al. Epidemiology of back pain in older adults: prevalence and risk factors for back pain onset. *Rheumatology (Oxford).* 2011;50(9):1645-1653.

4.Demyttenaere K, Bruffaerts R, Lee S, et al. Mental disorders among persons with chronic back or neck pain: results from the World Mental Health Surveys. *Pain.* 2007;129(3):332-342.

5.Qaseem A, Wilt TJ, McLean RM, Forciea MA, Clinical Guidelines Committee of the American College of P. Noninvasive Treatments for Acute, Subacute, and Chronic Low Back Pain: A Clinical Practice Guideline From the American College of Physicians. *Ann Intern Med.* 2017;166(7):514-530.

6.Summaries for patients. Physiotherapist-directed exercise, advice, or both for low back pain. *Ann Intern Med.* 2007;146(11):I56.

7.Hagen EM, Odelien KH, Lie SA, Eriksen HR. Adding a physical exercise programme to brief intervention for low back pain patients did not increase return to work. *Scand J Public Health.* 2010;38(7):731-738.

8.Machado LA, Maher CG, Herbert RD, Clare H, McAuley JH. The effectiveness of the McKenzie method in addition to first-line care for acute low back pain: a randomized controlled trial. *BMC Med.* 2010;8:10.

9.Rubinstein SM, Terwee CB, Assendelft WJ, de Boer MR, van Tulder MW. Spinal manipulative therapy for acute low-back pain. *Cochrane Database Syst Rev.* 2012(9):CD008880.

10.Rubinstein SM, Terwee CB, Assendelft WJ, de Boer MR, van Tulder MW. Spinal manipulative therapy for acute low back pain: an update of the cochrane review. *Spine (Phila Pa 1976).* 2013;38(3):E158-177.

11.Konczalik W, Elsayed S, Boszczyk B. Experience of a fellowship in spinal surgery: a quantitative analysis. *Eur Spine J.* 2014;23 Suppl 1:S40-54.

12.Grabel ZJ, Hart RA, Clark AP, et al. Adult Spinal Deformity Knowledge in Orthopedic Spine Surgeons: Impact of Fellowship Training, Experience, and Practice Characteristics. *Spine Deform.* 2018;6(1):60-66.

13.Clark AJ, Garcia RM, Keefe MK, et al. Results of the AANS membership survey of adult spinal deformity knowledge: impact of training, practice experience, and assessment of potential areas for improved education: Clinical article. *J Neurosurg Spine.* 2014;21(4):640-647.

14.Pejrona M, Ristori G, Villafane JH, Pregliasco FE, Berjano P. Does specialty matter? A survey on 176 Italian neurosurgeons and orthopedic spine surgeons confirms similar competency for common spinal conditions and supports multidisciplinary teams in comprehensive and complex spinal care. *Spine J.* 2017.

15.Boden SD. The use of radiographic imaging studies in the

evaluation of patients who have degenerative disorders of the lumbar spine. *J Bone Joint Surg Am.* 1996;78(1):114-124.

16.Boden SD, McCowin PR, Davis DO, Dina TS, Mark AS, Wiesel S. Abnormal magnetic-resonance scans of the cervical spine in asymptomatic subjects. A prospective investigation. *J Bone Joint Surg Am.* 1990;72(8):1178-1184.

www.ingramcontent.com/pod-product-compliance
Lightning Source LLC
Chambersburg PA
CBHW020155200326
41521CB00006B/376